"Taoist healing is based on the connection of energy flows of the universe and within the body. David Twicken presents a detailed description of the energy flows of the divergent channels and how to apply them in clinical practice. Twicken also presents a comprehensive ancient Taoist Nei Dan meditation to transform emotions into vitality and rejuvenating qi. The clinical applications and the Nei Dan practice are essential parts of Taoist healing. I highly recommend *The Divergent Channels—Jing Bie: A Handbook for Clinical Practice and Five Shen Nei Dan Inner Meditation* to healers of all traditions."

—*Taoist Grandmaster Mantak Chia, Founder of the Universal Healing Tao and Tao Garden, and author of* Healing Light of the Tao, Taoist Cosmic Healing, Awaken Healing Energy Through the Tao, *and* Chi Nei Tsang: Chi Massage for the Vital Organs

"Dr. David Twicken is one of the pre-eminent voices and teachers within American acupuncture. Part of his gifts lie in providing a clear context and explanation of classical Chinese medicine while providing practical clinical application. The results are treatments that are dynamic and flexible that aid patients in the transformation of their health conditions. I've had the great honor of learning directly under Dr. Twicken and the results of his treatment approaches, including divergent channel treatments, have been phenomenal. Patients have not only reported having significant improvement in chronic symptoms but also profound spiritual experiences that I haven't found with other treatment approaches."

—*Stephen Chee, M.D., Board-Certified Family Physician and Faculty at two Chinese Medicine programs*

"The divergent channels have fascinated acupuncturists for generations, but the medical classics offer little information beyond simple pathway descriptions and the admonition that they are important to know. In this text, David Twicken, an experienced practitioner of both Chinese medicine and Taoist (Daoist) inner alchemy, offers readers both a working clinical model of divergent channels and a window into his own deep exploration of these topics. Twicken also uses the clinical information as a jumping off point to describe the actual process of alchemy. This book challenges us to consider that there is much more to acupuncture practice than just the regular channels."

—*Dr. Henry McCann, DAOM, L.Ac., author of* Pricking the Vessels: Bloodletting Therapy in Chinese Medicine

"This is my new favorite of Dr. Twicken's many books displaying his masterful grasp of Taoist cycles, *I Ching*, and Chinese bio-psycho-spiritual medicine. It's a brilliant summary of how divergent channels integrate the 14 major treatment strategies and nine needling methods. He deciphers the complicated *Su Wen* and *Ling Shu* classics for us, with practical and elegant divergent strategies linking eight extra vessels/bone marrow, twelve organ meridians, muscle/tendon and skin levels. Especially valuable are four chapters on Nei Dan Five Shen, Cauldron and Orbit meditations that allow anyone to directly penetrate the psycho-energetic depths of their body's qi channels. Dr. Twicken has outdone himself. This fascinating book is a must-have for both healing professionals and Tao meditators seeking a lucid map of what's possible."

—*Michael Winn, co-author of seven books with Mantak Chia, author of ten nei dan homestudy courses, and Founder of Healing Tao University in North Carolina*

THE DIVERGENT CHANNELS
JING BIE

by the same author

Eight Extraordinary Channels—Qi Jing Ba Mai
A Handbook for Clinical Practice and Nei Dan Inner Meditation
ISBN 978 1 84819 148 8
eISBN 978 0 85701 137 4

I Ching Acupuncture—The Balance Method
Clinical Applications of the Ba Gua and I Ching
ISBN 978 1 84819 074 0
eISBN 978 0 85701 064 3

of related interest

Heavenly Streams
Meridian Theory in Nei Gong
Damo Mitchell
Foreword by Rob Aspell
ISBN 978 1 84819 116 7
eISBN 978 0 85701 092 6

The Compleat Acupuncturist
A Guide to Constitutional and Conditional Pulse Diagnosis
Peter Eckman
Foreword by William Morris
ISBN 978 1 84819 198 3
eISBN 978 0 85701 152 7

Heavenly Stems and Earthly Branches—TianGan DiZhi
The Heart of Chinese Wisdom Traditions
Master Zhongxian Wu and Dr. Karin Taylor Wu
Foreword by Fei BingXun
ISBN 978 1 84819 151 8
eISBN 978 0 85701 158 9

THE DIVERGENT CHANNELS
JING BIE

A Handbook for Clinical Practice and Five Shen Nei Dan Inner Meditation

DR. DAVID TWICKEN, DOM, L.AC.

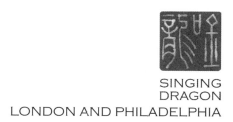

SINGING DRAGON
LONDON AND PHILADELPHIA

The figures in Chapters 1 and 4 are reprinted from Ni 1996 with kind permission from Yitian Ni and Complementary Medicine Press.
Figure 13.1 is reprinted with kind permission from Jerry Alan Johnson.
Figure 13.2 is reprinted with kind permission from Mantak Chia.

First published in 2014
by Singing Dragon
an imprint of Jessica Kingsley Publishers
73 Collier Street
London N1 9BE, UK
and
400 Market Street, Suite 400
Philadelphia, PA 19106, USA

www.singingdragon.com

Copyright © Dr. David Twicken, DOM, L.Ac. 2014

All rights reserved. No part of this publication may be reproduced in any material form (including photocopying or storing it in any medium by electronic means and whether or not transiently or incidentally to some other use of this publication) without the written permission of the copyright owner except in accordance with the provisions of the Copyright, Designs and Patents Act 1988 or under the terms of a licence issued by the Copyright Licensing Agency Ltd, Saffron House, 6–10 Kirby Street, London EC1N 8TS. Applications for the copyright owner's written permission to reproduce any part of this publication should be addressed to the publisher.

Warning: The doing of an unauthorised act in relation to a copyright work may result in both a civil claim for damages and criminal prosecution.

Library of Congress Cataloging in Publication Data
Twicken, David, author.
  The divergent channels - jing bie : a handbook for clinical practice and five shen nei dan inner meditation / Dr. David Twicken.
       p. ; cm.
  Jing bie
  Includes bibliographical references and index.
  ISBN 978-1-84819-189-1 (alk. paper)
  I. Title. II. Title: Jing bie.
  [DNLM: 1. Acupuncture Therapy--methods. 2. Medicine, Chinese Traditional--methods. 3. Meditation--methods. WB 369]
  RM184
  615.8'92--dc23
                            2014004227

British Library Cataloguing in Publication Data
A CIP catalogue record for this book is available from the British Library

ISBN 978 1 84819 189 1
eISBN 978 0 85701 150 3

Printed and bound in Great Britain by Bell & Bain Ltd, Glasgow

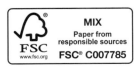

CONTENTS

Disclaimer 11
Acknowledgments 12
Author Note 13
Chinese Dynasties 15

Introduction 17

PART I BACKGROUND

1 The Divergent Channels Pathways 27
2 Working It Out 43
3 Divergent Channels Sequencing Theories 47
4 The Divergent Channels 67

PART II WORKING IT OUT

5 The Major and Connecting Channels 89
6 Cycles of Time 101
7 The Five Shen 113
8 The Nine Needles 131
9 Guiding Theories and Principles 141

PART III CLINICAL APPLICATIONS

10 The Clinical Applications of Divergent Channels Theory . . 155

PART IV NEI DAN INNER MEDITATION

11 Introduction to Nei Dan Inner Meditation 173

12 The Cauldron 183

13 The Small Heavenly Orbit 187

14 Five Shen Nei Dan Inner Meditation 197

Conclusion 213

Endnotes 214
Bibliography 216
Index 217

LIST OF FIGURES AND TABLES

Figures

3.1	The He Tu diagram	48
3.2	The He Tu diagram with numbers	49
3.3	The He Tu and the five phases	51
3.4	The Early Heaven Ba Gua	53
3.5	The Ba Gua and their positions	54
3.6	The Ba Gua and their positions and strokes	55
3.7	The structure of the Early Heaven Ba Gua	56
3.8	The Ba Gua and the channels	63
6.1	The meridian clock	102
7.1	The five shen	126
8.1	The nine needles	134
11.1	The three dan tian	178
13.1	The lower dan tian	188
13.2	The small heavenly orbit	191
14.1	The collection points	206

Tables

3.1	The eight trigrams and the channels	64
4.1	The divergent channels main points	83
4.2	Roots and ends	85
5.1	The connecting channel pathology	98
6.1	The muscle channels and the twelve lunar months	104
6.2	The wei qi and the muscle channels cycle	105
6.3	The hour stem and branch table	111
7.1	Five shen and correspondences	130
8.1	Nine needles summary	137
8.2	The nine needles and the channels of acupuncture	138
8.3	The nine needles and the channels and conditions	138
9.1	Roots and ends	147
10.1	The divergent channels' confluent and pathway points	170
14.1	Five phases correspondences	198

DISCLAIMER

The information in this book is based on the author's knowledge and personal experience. This information is presented for educational purposes to assist the reader in expanding his or her knowledge of Chinese philosophy and Chinese medicine. The techniques and practices are to be used at the reader's own discretion and liability. The author is not responsible in any manner whatsoever for any physical injury that may occur by following instructions in this book.

ACKNOWLEDGMENTS

I would like to give a special thank you to Master Mantak Chia for sharing Qi Gong, meditation, internal alchemy, and Taoism with compassion, respect, and love. I would also like to thank him for the illustration in Figure 13.2.

Thank you, Yitian Ni and Complementary Medicine Press, for the illustrations in Chapters 1 and 4.

Thank you, Jerry Alan Johnson, for the illustration in Figure 13.1.

Thank you, Gregory E. Leblanc, L.Ac., Dr. Fritz Hudnut, DAOM, L.Ac., Jennifer Minor, Michael Winn, Steven Sy, and Marika Chandler, L.Ac., for your editing contributions.

Thank you, Jessica Kingsley and your excellent team at Singing Dragon, for all your work in publishing this book.

AUTHOR NOTE

The beauty of Chinese philosophy, metaphysics, and the healing arts is they are based on a unified view of life. Chinese medicine is applied philosophy. It is applying the insights of the ancient Chinese philosophers, astronomers, and shaman healers to the human body. Century after century, philosophical and practical knowledge accumulated based on trial and error, culminating in a sophisticated and profound natural healing system. I have attempted to retain the insight of the Han dynasty classics, the *Su Wen* and the *Ling Shu*, as the philosophical and clinical source for applying the divergent channels in practice. This book is based on three aspects of my experiences. The first is 30 years of studying Chinese philosophy, including Chinese metaphysics, *I Ching*, Chinese astrology, feng shui, qi men dun jia, nei dan, Qi Gong, and the Chinese calendar. The second is more than two decades of clinical experience. And the third is teaching theory and clinical applications to students and interns at Chinese medical schools.

There are five major acupuncture channels in the acupuncture system. They are the muscle, connecting, primary, separate (divergent), and the eight extraordinary channels. The divergent channels are unique in that they link or connect to all of the channel systems. A main goal of this book is to present *Ling Shu* and *Su Wen* theories and applications to show how the divergent channels can treat all the channels. There are a few translations of the words *Jing Bie*, some of which are separate channels, divergent channels, channel divergences, the distinct channels, and the reticular channels. From these I have chosen to use the names "separate channels" or "divergent channels"; I don't feel the translation influences the clinical applications. Learning theory and functions of the channels guide clinical applications.

This book is designed to present theories and clinical applications. There should be a seamless line between understanding and application. This understanding builds intention, and a fluidity of thought and action. Based on knowledge, application, and intention, we become not only technically proficient practitioners, but artists in the way we perceive and devise unique treatment plans for each patient. This is the essence of Chinese medicine.

This book is part of a series of books on Chinese medicine, and the life arts that contribute to understanding the foundation theories of the ancient healers, and how to apply their insights in modern life.

CHINESE DYNASTIES

Dynasty	Years
Pre-historic period	
Yangshao	5000 BC
Longshan	2500 BC
Xia	2100–1600 BC
Historic period	
Shang	1600–1045 BC
Zhou	1045–221 BC
Western Zhou	1045–771 BC
Eastern Zhou	770–256 BC
Spring and Autumn Period	722–481 BC
Warring States Period	403–221 BC
Qin	221–206 BC
Han	206 BC–AD 220
Western Han	206 BC–AD 24
Eastern Han	25 AD–AD 220
Three Kingdoms	220–280
Jin (Western and Eastern)	265–420
Southern and Northern	420–589
Sui	581–618
Tang	618–907
Five Dynasties and Ten Kingdoms	907–960

Song	960–1279
Liao	916–1125
Jin	1115–1234
Yuan	1271–1368
Ming	1368–1644
Qing (Manchu)	1644–1911
Republic of China	1912–1949
People's Republic of China	1949–present

INTRODUCTION

As a teenager I remember gazing out of my window on a cold winter night in New Hampshire, the stars shining bright, the moon seeming so close I could reach out and touch it. I had a sense that answers to my questions about the nature of life would include a deep understanding of the stars, planets, and cycles of nature. During the next three decades I studied Chinese philosophy and the Chinese healing and life arts. Chinese philosophy includes Yin–Yang, five phases, eight trigrams, the Ba Gua, He Tu, Nine Palaces Luo Shu, celestial stems, terrestrial branches, and the Chinese calendar. The healing and life arts include feng shui, Chinese astrology, *I Ching*, Qi Gong, nei dan, Tai Chi Chuan, qi men dun jia, acupuncture, and herbal medicine. These arts contain the fundamental theories and principles that comprise a primary aspect of the Han dynasty Chinese medical classics: the *Su Wen* and the *Ling Shu*.

The early practitioners of Chinese medicine perceived the resonance between nature and humanity. They studied astronomy in depth. They mapped out the sky and the locations and movements of the planets and stars. This was the cosmic map. They turned their focus internally and perceived the energy fields within the human body, and mapped out the human body. This was the inner map of the body. This map is a magnificent, detailed, and comprehensive guide to the structure and functioning of the body. In the early Chinese medical classic texts—the *Su Wen, Ling Shu, Pulse Classic*, and the *Classic of Acupuncture and Moxibustion*— the inner map of the human body is presented in detail. This map contains the acupuncture system:

- Cutaneous channels
- Muscle (sinew) channels
- Connecting (luo) channels
- Primary (major) channels
- Divergent (separate) channels
- Eight extraordinary channels

Chapter 27 of the *Su Wen* captures the ancients' insight into the relationship between nature and humanity:

> A well-rounded physician must have a certain set of principles in medicine and must also observe the changes in nature. For example, in the heavens there are changes in the positions of the sun, the moon with its waxing and waning, and the constellations. On the earth there are rivers, tributaries, and oceans. In human beings there are the channels and collaterals. These influence each other. When the weather warms, the flow of waters in the rivers becomes calm and easy. When the weather is cold, the flow of waters stagnates. When the weather is excessively hot, however, the waters in the rivers become abundant, and flooding results. If the storms begin, further disasters occur. Similarly, an external pathogen invades the body. Cold causes the channels and collateral blood and qi to stagnate. Heat will cause blood to flow very freely and rapidly. Excessive heat will cause the channels and collaterals to swell.[1]

This *Su Wen* passage expresses how patterns and interactions in nature were perceived as mirrors of the interactions in the human body. The early contributors of Chinese philosophy and medicine saw a deep parallel between nature and humanity, and they expressed their insights in many ways in classic books. Some correspondences are uniquely presented in Chapter 71 of the *Ling Shu*, "The Mutual Resonance between Heaven, Human, and Earth":[2]

- Heaven is round and Earth is flat. A human's head is round and the feet are flat.

- Heaven has the sun and moon. Humans have two eyes.
- Earth has nine regions. Humans have nine orifices.
- Heaven has wind and rain. Humans have joy and anger.
- Heaven has four seasons. Humans have four limbs.
- Heaven has the five tones. Humans have five viscera.
- Heaven has winter and summer. Humans have chills and fever.
- Heaven has the ten celestial stems. Humans have ten fingers.
- Heaven has Yin and Yang. Humans have male and female.
- The year has 365 days. Humans have 365 sections.
- Earth has high mountains. Humans have shoulders and kneecaps.
- Earth has deep valleys. Humans have armpits and creases of the knees.
- Heaven has day and night. Humans have waking and sleeping.
- Heaven has stars. Humans have teeth.
- Earth has small hills. Humans have small joints.
- Earth has stony mountains. Humans have prominent bones.
- Earth has forest and trees. Humans have muscles.
- Earth has an accumulation of cities. Humans have accumulations of flesh at major joints.
- The year has twelve months. Humans have twelve major joints.
- Earth has springs and streams. Humans have protective qi.
- Earth has twelve rivers. Humans have twelve major channels.

Correspondences are relationships. Perceiving relationships between the environment and the human body is an essential aspect of Chinese medicine. The observation of the external environment led to a deep observation of the internal environment, and the inner map of the human body was revealed. The early Chinese philosophies (for example, Yin–Yang and the five phases) were applied to the human body to understand and explain the relationships inside the body. For centuries, the internal functions and relationships were studied and a comprehensive system of natural medicine developed. Chinese medicine is a deep study of these interactions and relationships. And the inner map of the human body reveals a complex structure and function of the body, mind, and spirit. It is in this structure and function that the clinical applications of the divergent channels is uncovered.

Chinese medicine and the acupuncture channel system include the influences of time and space. Time includes the movements of the sun, the moon, and all the planets. It also includes cycles of time, especially year, season, month, and day cycles. These cycles have energetic influences on the body. The early classics of acupuncture present these cycles and their influences. The acupuncture channels are the spaces where the energetic influences of time manifest.

Space includes the earth and its terrain. The waterways in our environment are an important image used in Chinese medicine. The five transporting points—well, spring, stream, river, and sea points—are an example of the correspondences of nature and the human body. The waterways flow in nature, and the early practitioners of Chinese medicine perceived that there were flows of vital substance in the body. Chinese medicine includes a deep study of how these vital substances flow in patterns and spaces throughout the body. The divergent channels have a powerful relationship and influence on vital substances, spaces, and cycles of time.

The Chinese medical classics present how pathogens can transfer throughout the channel system (the spaces of the body). Pathogens and imbalances include the six exogenous factors, and the seven emotions. The six exogenous pathogenic factors are wind, cold, damp, heat, summer heat, and dryness. The seven emotions are anger, joy, sadness, grief, pensiveness, fear, and fright. Understanding where pathogens are located is essential in developing effective treatment plans. The following references from the *Su Wen* and the *Ling Shu* present the layers of the body. This layering is the foundation for making a diagnosis and a treatment plan:

> It is said the illness may be on the hair level, the skin level, the muscle level, the level of channels, the tendon level, and bone and marrow level. When treating the hair level do not damage the skin level. If the illness is at the skin level do not damage the muscle level, if the illness is at the muscle level needling too deeply will damage the channel level. In illness of the tendons needling too deeply will damage the bone level, in illness of the bones needling too deeply will damage the marrow.[3]

> Don't just stare at disease. Begin by knowing which channels are diseased. For illness, know its origins. First know which channels are diseased, then treat them at those locations.[4]

These *Su Wen* and *Ling Shu* references guide the practitioner to a very important principle: a diagnosis should include the channels affected by the condition. Knowing where the condition is located (the channel system) provides the foundation for developing a targeted treatment plan, which is essential for an effective treatment.

Chapter 5 of the *Ling Shu*, "Roots and Ends," offers a unique insight into the function of the divergent channels:

> There are an extraordinary number of diseases in the separate (divergent) channels. They cannot be counted without knowing the roots and ends of the five viscera and six bowels. Disease can break open the gates and upset the pivots and travel through the gates and inner doors.[5]

This quote can be interpreted as meaning that the divergent channels are an integral part of the acupuncture channel system, and pathology and imbalances within the body can be transferred into these channels. Therefore, pathogens throughout the body can transfer into the divergent channels. This total body connection explains how there can be an extraordinary number of diseases in the divergent channels. This connection is the reason why the divergent channels can treat all the channels of acupuncture.

The divergent channels can treat any channel system alone, or they can be used along with other channel systems. For example, if there is chronic Liver fire, the Liver and Gallbladder divergent channels can be treated alone to release the Liver fire. In that same condition, the Liver and Gallbladder primary channels can be added to the treatment (the Liver and Gallbladder connecting channels could be treated as well). A synergy can occur when two or more channels or channel systems are combined; the result is often better than using one channel. The effects of mobilizing the energies of the entire body are essential in effective treatments. The ability of the divergent channels to assist all the channel systems is an important quality of the divergent channels.

The divergent channels are presented in Chapter 11 of the *Ling Shu*. The chapter is called "The Separate Channels." This is the only chapter in the *Ling Shu* that presents the divergent channels; however, only the pathways of the divergent channels are presented. The *Su Wen* and the *Nan Ching* do not mention them. The Jin dynasty classic book, *The Classic of Acupuncture and Moxibustion (Jia Yi Jing)*, basically presents the information found in the *Ling Shu*. Throughout the long history of Chinese medicine, there is very little written about the divergent channels in medical texts.

In Chapter 11 of the *Ling Shu*, "The Separate Channels," there is unique advice about the divergent channels:

> Study these first. Work it out to the finish. The unskilled think it is easy; the superior know it is difficult. Please explain these separations and joinings, these exits and entrances. The skilled pass right by them, while they are the very breath of the superior physician.[6]

The goal of this book is to *work it out*. This book contains theories, interpretations, and clinical applications based on working out the insights of the ancient Chinese philosophers, cosmologists, and *Su Wen* and *Ling Shu* practitioners. Each chapter presents an important element in working out the theory and reasoning for the clinical applications of the divergent channels. The applications presented in this book have been applied in my clinical practice. I have also guided interns in their clinical applications as a clinic supervisor. I have found the divergent channels to be one of the most useful and effective channel systems in clinical practice.

This book includes a special nei dan cultivation: *Five Shen Nei Dan*. It is also called *Fusion of the Five Phases*. Nei dan is inner meditation, a type of inner cultivation of the three treasures: jing, qi, and shen. It is a profound way to transform your emotions and conditioning which has become your constitution. This nei dan is based on the traditional information you learn about the five phases, including the colors, organs, elements, shen, temperatures, and the climate that relates to each of them. These correspondences of the five phases are cultivated to allow the natural, innate virtues each of us is endowed with to shine bright in our life. This is an ancient Taoist meditation that can assist in your life path. It is based on Chapter 5 of the *Su Wen*, "The Manifestation of Yin and Yang from the Macrocosm to the Microcosm," and Chapter 8 of the *Ling Shu*, "The Roots of Spirit." In my experience as a meditator and teacher, it is a powerful meditation for emotional transformation.

The early developers of Chinese medicine left a path for future practitioners. The path of the ancient doctors is found in the classics and in their clinical experience. The early philosophers and medical practitioners left profound theories, models, and tools to understand a changing world. Part of our journey as practitioners is to trace the path of these extraordinary people. Tracing the path includes a deep study of Chinese metaphysics. This knowledge contributes towards us becoming medical thinkers, and developing the ability to respond to changing environments.

The divergent channels may be the most flexible of all the channel systems. They provide the opportunity to gather the body's resources to treat a condition, creating a healing synergy. This is holistic healing, the essence of Chinese medicine. I wrote this book with the primary objective of presenting a clear, practical handbook for applying the divergent channels in clinical practice. I hope you enjoy it and find it helpful in your practice.

Part I

BACKGROUND

CHAPTER 1

THE DIVERGENT CHANNELS PATHWAYS

> Study these first. Work it out to the finish. The unskilled think it is easy; the superior know it is difficult. Please explain these separations and joinings, these exits and entrances. The skilled pass right by them, while they are the very breath of the superior physician.[7]

The pathways of the acupuncture channel system create the inner map of the body. These pathways are the space where vital substances (jing, qi, blood, and body fluids) are distributed. They also are the locations where pathogens can be lodged. Learning the pathways is the key to understanding how to apply the divergent channels in clinical practice. Chapter 11 of the *Ling Shu*, "The Separate Channels," presents the divergent channels pathways. The first presentation in this book is directly from the *Ling Shu*; drawings have been added for a clear image of them. Chapter 4 includes common points along the pathways with an example of how to use the channels in clinical practice. Both the drawings and points are information added to the original information in the *Ling Shu*. "The Separate Channels" in the *Ling Shu* does not include any pathology for the divergent channels.

The original presentation of the divergent channels from the *Ling Shu* provides clarity of their path throughout the body. The path reveals intersections and relationships within the body. Knowing the locations through which the pathways flow provides the base for evaluating the common theories and clinical applications in the acupuncture community. This knowledge can guide you on how to apply the divergent channels in clinical practice.

The first goal in learning about the divergent channels is to have a clear understanding of their internal pathways. Pathogens can lodge in areas along the pathways. The areas where the divergent pathways connect, cross, or converge with other channels have a dual influence. First, pathogens from other channels can transfer into the divergent channels at these intersection areas. Second, the divergent channels can influence these areas. By treating these intersections, we can influence the entire body. For example, wind-damp-cold in the lower back can transfer to the middle and upper spine. The Bladder divergent channel flows along the spine. The Bladder divergent channel can be treated to clear the pathogen from the spine, and the Kidney divergent channel can assist in helping the Bladder divergent channel clear the pathogen. The Du channel could also be used to assist the treatment. Understanding the pathways and their interactions with other channels and anatomical areas is an essential aspect in applying the divergent channels in clinical practice.

THE DIVERGENT CHANNELS PATHWAYS
First junction (confluence)
BLADDER AND KIDNEY DIVERGENT CHANNELS

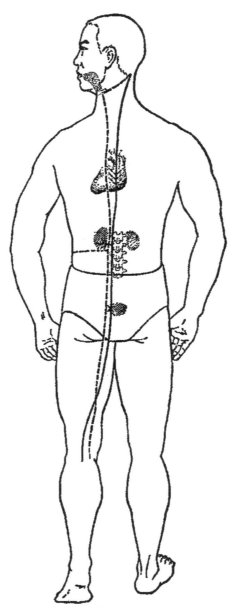

Bladder divergent channel (—)
Kidney divergent channel (---)

Bladder divergent channel

The separate channel of the primary Leg Major Yang separates from the popliteal fossa of the knee. A branch goes to a point five cun below the hip joint, and branches to enter the anus. It connects with the Bladder, spreads to the Kidneys, and then follows along and to the sides of the spine and spreads in the region of the Heart. Branches follow the backbone up, come out in the neck, and again connect with the Major Yang. Here they join and make one channel.

Kidney divergent channel

The separate channel of the primary Leg Minor Yin connects to the popliteal fossa of the knee, separates and joins the Major Yang, and then goes up to reach the Kidneys. At the fourteenth vertebra, the second lumbar, it comes out and connects to the girdle channel. A branch connects with the root of the tongue and comes out in the neck, *where it joins the Major Yang to make the first junction.*

Second junction (confluence)
GALLBLADDER AND LIVER DIVERGENT CHANNELS

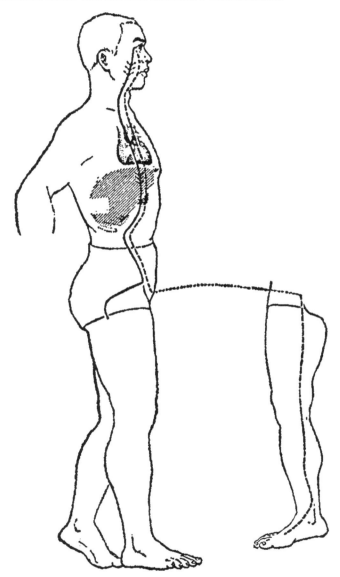

Gallbladder divergent channel (—)
Liver divergent channel (---)

Gallbladder divergent channel

The separate channel of the primary Leg Minor Yang winds around the thigh and enters the border of the pubic hair margin to join the Shrinking Yin channel. A branch enters the lowest ribs and follows the base of the diaphragm to connect to the Gallbladder. It then spreads to the top of the Liver, passes through the Heart, to the throat to come out at the chin and jaw to spread into the face. It connects with the eye, and then joins the Minor Yang at the lateral corner of the eye.

Liver divergent channel

The separate channel of the primary Leg Shrinking Yin separates at the top of the foot, and ascends to the pubic hair, where it joins the Minor Yang. *There they travel together and make the second junction.*

Third junction (confluence)
STOMACH AND SPLEEN DIVERGENT CHANNELS

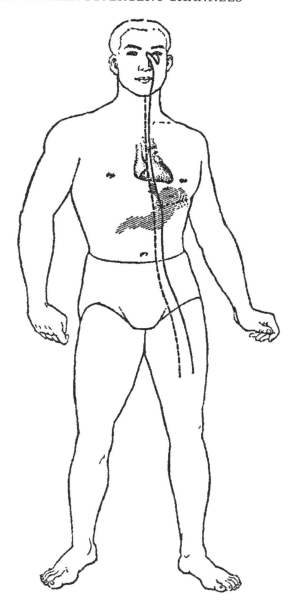

Stomach divergent channel (—)
Spleen divergent channel (---)

Stomach divergent channel

The separate channel of the primary Leg Bright Yang ascends to reach the thigh, enters into the base of the abdomen, and connects to the Stomach. It then spreads to the Spleen, ascends and penetrates the Heart. It flows to the throat to come out in the mouth, then continues up to the nose and forehead to pass through and connect with the eye, and joins in the Rushing Yang.

Spleen divergent channel

The primary Leg Major Yin ascends to reach the buttocks, where it joins the Rushing Yang. Together, ascend to connect in the throat, and pass through the middle (root) of the tongue. *This makes the third junction.*

Fourth junction (confluence)
SMALL INTESTINE AND HEART DIVERGENT CHANNELS

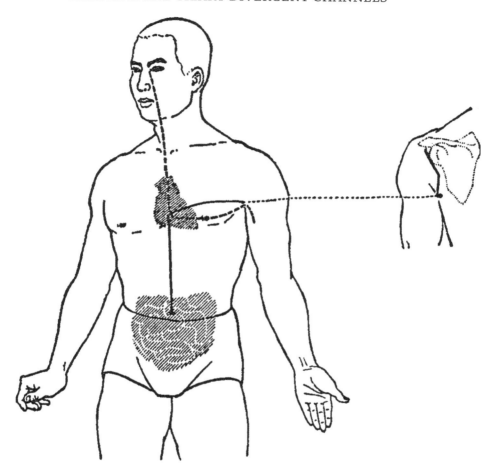

Small Intestine divergent channel (—)
Heart divergent channel (---)

Small Intestine divergent channel

The separate channel of the primary Arm Major Yang separates from the scapula to enter the armpit, reaches the Heart, and connects to the Small Intestine.

Heart divergent channel

The separate channel of the primary Arm Minor Yin enters the point between two tendons to enter the Abyss of the Armpit and links to the Heart. It ascends to the throat, and then comes out in the face. *There it joins the Major Yang at the medial corner of the eye (inner canthus) and makes the fourth junction.*

Fifth junction (confluence)
SAN JIAO AND PERICARDIUM DIVERGENT CHANNELS

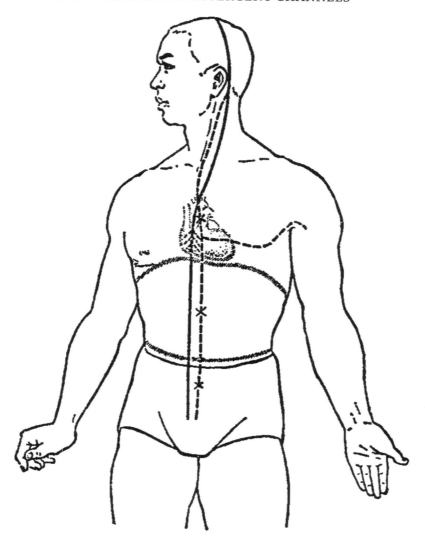

San Jiao divergent channel (—)
Pericardium divergent channel (---)

San Jiao divergent channel

The separate channel of the primary Arm Minor Yang descends from the top of the head to enter the supraclavicular fossa (Broken Dish) and it descends through the Triple Heater and scatters in the middle of the chest.

Pericardium divergent channel

The separate channel of the primary Arm Shrinking Yin channel separates three cun below the Abyss of the Armpit and enters the center of the chest, where it separates to link to the Triple Heater. It runs along the throat, and then comes out behind the ear. It joins the Minor Yang below the Final Bone. *This makes the fifth junction.*

THE DIVERGENT CHANNELS PATHWAYS

Sixth junction (confluence)
LARGE INTESTINE AND LUNG DIVERGENT CHANNELS

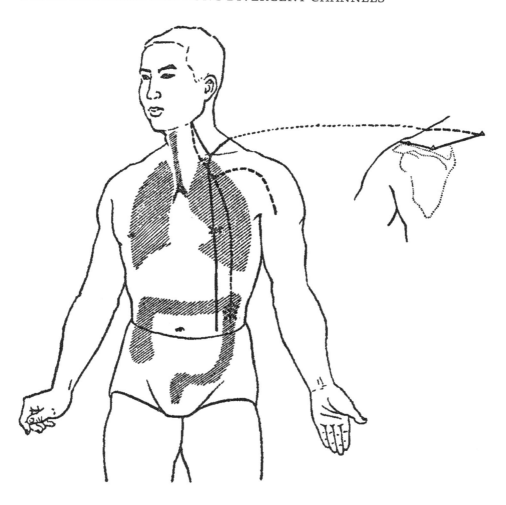

Large Intestine divergent channel (—)
Lung divergent channel (---)

Large Intestine divergent channel

The separate channel of the primary Arm Bright Yang flows from the hand to the chest and breast. There it separates to go to the Shoulder Bone and enters the Pillar Bone. It descends and links to the Large Intestine. It connects to the Lungs, flows along the throat, and comes out in the Broken Dish to join the Bright Yang.

Lung divergent channel

The separate channel of the primary Arm Major Yin separates and passes the Abyss of the Armpit in front of the Minor Yin, and then links to the Lungs. It flows to the Large Intestine and ascends to the Broken Dish, flows along the throat, and then returns to join the Arm Bright Channel. *This makes the sixth junction.*

THE DIVERGENT CHANNELS SEQUENCE

The following channel order is how the divergent channels are presented in the *Ling Shu*. However, the order does not follow any of the standard models in Chinese medical theory. For example, the order of the channels does not follow the creation or the controlling cycle of the five phases. It does not follow the nourishing qi cycle (daily meridian clock) or the six-stage cycle: Tai Yang, Yang Ming, Shao Yang, Tai Yin, Shao Yin, and Jue Yin. This chapter and the following chapter of this book present classic Chinese philosophical models that support the sequence of the divergent channels.

Foot channels
FIRST JUNCTION (UNION, CONFLUENCE)

- Foot Tai Yang and Foot Shao Yin
- Bladder and Kidney channels
- Water element

Second junction (union, confluence)

- Foot Shao Yang and Foot Jue Yin
- Gallbladder and Liver channels
- Wood element

Third junction (union, confluence)

- Foot Yang Ming and Foot Tai Yin
- Stomach and Spleen channels
- Earth element

Hand channels

Fourth junction (union, confluence)

- Hand Tai Yang and Hand Shao Yin
- Small Intestine and Heart channels
- Fire element

Fifth junction (union, confluence)

- Hand Shao Yang and Hand Jue Yin
- San Jiao and Pericardium channels
- Fire element

Sixth junction (union, confluence)

- Hand Yang Ming and Hand Tai Yin
- Large Intestine and Lung channels
- Metal element

Analysis of the divergent channels sequence

The divergent channels are presented in the following elemental pattern: water, wood, earth, fire, fire, and metal. This pattern follows the distribution of the primary channels along the leg and arm. This is the *space* aspect of time and space. The divergent channels begin on the foot with a Yang channel and flow in the following pattern: Tai Yang, Shao Yang, and Yang Ming. Beginning with the Foot Tai Yang channel (Bladder), and moving in a Yang pattern, which is to the lateral aspect of the body, the Foot Shao Yang (Gallbladder) channel follows. The next Foot Yang channel is located at the front of the foot. This channel is the Foot Yang Ming (Stomach) channel. These are the three Foot Yang channels. They are also the water, wood, and earth elements. The order of this flow is space or location based.

The second set of channel patterns are the Foot Yin channels. They are the Yin–Yang pairs of the set of channels just presented. The distribution of these channels is on the medial (Yin) aspect of the foot. The first is the Foot Shao Yin channel. This is the Kidney channel. It is the Yin–Yang pair of the Foot Tai Yang channel, the Bladder. The pair is the Bladder and the Kidneys. This is the Foot Tai Yang and the Foot Shao Yin pair. The second channel in the pattern is the Yin–Yang pair of the Foot Shao Yang. It is the Foot Jue Yin channel, the Liver. The Foot Shao Yang and the Foot Jue Yin are Yin–Yang pairs. The third channel is the Yin–Yang pair of the Foot Yang Ming channel. It is the Spleen. The Stomach and the Spleen are Yin–Yang pairs.

The hand divergent channels follow the same pattern. The Yang pattern is the Hand Tai Yang, the Small Intestine; the Hand Shao Yang, the San Jiao; and the Hand Yang Ming, the Large Intestine. The paired Yin channels are the Heart, the Pericardium, and the Lung. From the six-channel viewpoint, they are the Hand Shao Yin, the Hand Jue Yin, and the Hand Tai Yin. The element pattern is fire, fire, and metal.

The channel distribution of the divergent channels throughout the body is the pattern Tai Yang, Shao Yang, and Yang Ming. The paired Yin channels follow that pattern. There are two classic Chinese energetic models and theories that support this sequence. The first is the He Tu, and the second is the Early Heaven Ba Gua. These two ancient diagrams and their theories are presented in Chapter 3.

CHAPTER 2

WORKING IT OUT

The *Ling Shu* advises that the practitioner should *work it out* to understand the functions and clinical applications of the divergent channels. In this chapter, the process of working it out begins, providing the guiding theories and principles for clinical applications of the divergent channels. The clinical applications will be based on the following insight of the *Ling Shu* practitioners, and the seven aspects of Chinese medicine presented below.

The *Ling Shu*, Chapter 5, "Roots and Ends," states:

> There are an extraordinary number of diseases in the separate (divergent) channels. They cannot be counted without knowing the roots and ends of the five organs and six bowels. Diseases can break open the gates and upset the pivots and travel through the gates and inner doors.[8]

Tracing the roots (beginnings) and ends (endings) of the five organs and the six bowels reveals how the anatomical regions, channels, organs, and pathogens can be transferred into the divergent channels. These patterns or connections also reveal that the divergent channels can treat pathogens or pathology in all the related connections (locations). This integrated web flows both ways. Each part of the channel network can influence the other. Imbalances can flow into the divergent channels, and imbalances in the divergent channels can flow to the channels they are connected with. Because the channels and body are integrated, an *extraordinary number of diseases* can be transferred from all over the body into the divergent channels. The divergent channels are connected to the superficial layer, which includes the sinew and connecting channels; the middle layer, which includes the primary channels and the internal organs; and the deep layer, which includes the eight extraordinary channels. Thus imbalances in those channels can transfer into the divergent channels. In other words, conditions located in the wei, ying, and yuan layers of the body can be transferred in the divergent channels.

The following list of seven qualities and relationships within the acupuncture system provides the basis for applying divergent channels in clinical practice. These Chinese medical qualities are from the *Ling Shu*, also known as *The Spiritual Pivot (Spiritual Compass)*. The *Ling Shu* is the compass that guides us to clinical applications of the divergent channels:

1. The divergent channels treat conditions along their pathways. The divergent channels include locations where the primary channels are not located. Understanding the divergent channels pathways is essential for clinical practice.

2. The divergent channels treat their associated internal organs. The divergent channels begin and end on the primary channels, and either the Yin or the Yang pair divergent channel connects to their related internal organs. These relationships directly influence the internal organs.

3. The divergent channels can treat conditions of their related primary channels. The divergent channels treat the primary channel's conditions found in Chapter 10 of the *Ling Shu*, "The Major Channels." When there are pathogenic factors in the primary channels (in this situation, not the internal organs), the divergent channels can assist in treating the condition.

4. The divergent channels can treat conditions of their related connecting (luo) channels. Chapter 10 of the *Ling Shu*, "The Major Channels," presents information about the connecting channels. The divergent channels can treat the connecting (luo) channels, especially emotional conditions related to the connecting channels.

5. The divergent channels can treat conditions of the muscle (sinew) channels. Chapter 13 of the *Ling Shu*, "The Muscle Channels," describes the muscle channels and their pathologies.

6. The divergent channels treat conditions found in the *Ling Shu*, Chapter 14, "Measurements in Reference to the Bones." Bones are connected to muscles, tendons, the eight extraordinary channels, and jing. The divergent channels can treat conditions in the eight extraordinary channels and jing.

7. The *Ling Shu* chapters before and after the separate (divergent) channels chapter offer clues for clinical applications. In addition to the chapters just listed, Chapter 5, "Roots and Ends," Chapter 8, "The Roots and Spirit," Chapter 9, "From Beginning to End," Chapter 12, "Rivers and Channels," Chapter 15, "The Fifty Regulators," and Chapter 16, "The Nourishing Qi," can be referenced to provide the framework for understanding clinical applications of the divergent channels.

These seven facets of Chinese medicine provide the foundation for divergent channels theory and clinical applications. Chapters 5 through 9 of this book are the *working it out* chapters. These chapters include explanations of the relationships between Chinese medical theories and principles, and the divergent channels. They provide a model for applying the divergent channels in clinical practice.

CHAPTER 3

DIVERGENT CHANNELS SEQUENCING THEORIES

The ancient Chinese developed unique ways to express insights they perceived about the environment. They studied the sun and the moon and the effects of these on their life. They felt the influences of the seasons and made detailed descriptions of the effects of these on their body and mind. Based on the study of nature, four ancient energy models developed in China contain many of the theories and principles in the *Su Wen* and the *Ling Shu*. The models are the He Tu, the Luo Shu, and the Early Heaven and the Later Heaven Ba Gua. See the author's book, *I Ching Acupuncture—The Balance Method* (Twicken 2011), for a detailed explanation of them. The theories of the He Tu and the Early Heaven Ba Gua support the distribution sequence of the divergent channels. Both of these models are now presented.

THE HE TU

The He Tu is a profound diagram with applications in many Chinese arts. The He Tu contains guiding principles that are found in the *I Ching*, the *Su Wen*, and *Ling Shu* theory. This chapter presents important principles contained in this ancient diagram.

According to Chinese legend, Fu Xi found the He Tu diagram during prehistoric times. The origin is unknown. We do know it is a very old diagram, which probably originated during early Chinese culture. The essence of its meaning was not commonly known until the legendary *I Ching* master, Shao Yong, analyzed it during the Song dynasty. Shao Yong did what now seems like an obvious thing: he converted the He Tu dots into a number system. Shao Yong counted the dots and assigned Yang to odd numbers, and Yin to even numbers. Additionally, he noticed that dark dots are Yin, and light dots are Yang. Shao Yong combined these two patterns to reveal that the He Tu contained a code: odd numbers and light dots are Yang, and even numbers and dark dots are Yin. Figure 3.1 presents the He Tu.

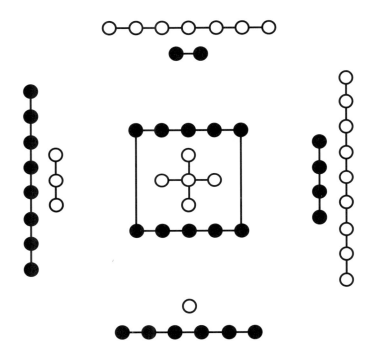

Figure 3.1 The He Tu diagram

The He Tu has a number system: count the dots to find their number. Dark dots are Yin, and light dots are Yang. Figure 3.2 shows the ancient number system of the He Tu.

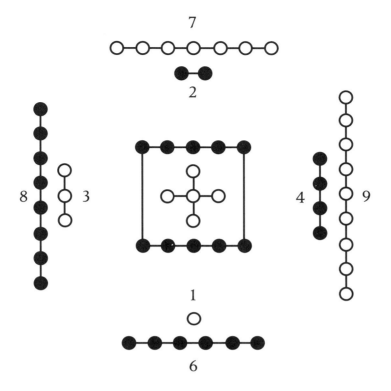

Figure 3.2 The He Tu diagram with numbers

One essential principle in the He Tu is that each of the four directions has a pair; nothing is in isolation. Notice that each area, the top and the bottom, and the left and the right, contains two sets of numbers. Each area contains the fundamental principle of Yin–Yang: there is an odd or Yang number, and an even or Yin number. Additionally, there are light dots and dark dots in each direction, which represent Yang and Yin. These relationships are the basis of a guiding principle: all things in life contain Yin and Yang.

The five phases were identified within the He Tu. The five phases creation cycle was placed over the diagram. The bottom of the He Tu is water, the left is wood, the top is fire, the right is metal, and the center is earth.

It is believed that the He Tu diagram predates Yin–Yang theory, but contains the principles of Yin–Yang. In the He Tu diagram there are eight directions or areas grouped into four sets of two pairs. This grouping is the guiding principle for pairing areas of the body and the acupuncture channels. For example, the limbs contain correspondences or pairs: the ankle and wrist; the knee and elbow; and the hip and shoulder. Because these anatomical structures are pairs, they treat each other. For example, for conditions at the wrist, treat the ankle. The He Tu contains the seeds of the eventual grouping of the twelve acupuncture channels into six pairs of channels: the Yin–Yang pairs.

In each of the cardinal directions there are two numbers: one is an odd number, which is Yang, and one is an even number, which is Yin, reflecting Yin–Yang in each direction. At the center there are five dots. Five represents the center. Five is also the earth element, and this diagram reveals that all elements, numbers, and directions originate in the center (earth). Each He Tu combination is related to the number five: $6 - 1 = 5$; $9 - 4 = 5$; $8 - 3 = 5$; and $7 - 2 = 5$. All these combinations originate from the center of the He Tu. In the He Tu, the center is earth and reflects the Spleen and Stomach. Each of the four pairs has a difference of the number five, which is the center. Each of the directional numbers shares an element: 1, 6 combine to create water; 2, 7 combine to create fire; 3, 8 combine to create wood; and 4, 9 combine to create metal. The Yin–Yang paired numbers and directions are the basis for the guest and host acupuncture treatments. "Guest and host" means combining Yin–Yang paired channels in a treatment. Combining the Large Intestine and the Lungs in a treatment, or combining the Spleen and Stomach in a treatment, are examples of a guest and host treatment. Chapter 9 of the *Ling Shu*, "From Beginning to End," presents using Yin–Yang pairs in treatments.

Structure of the He Tu

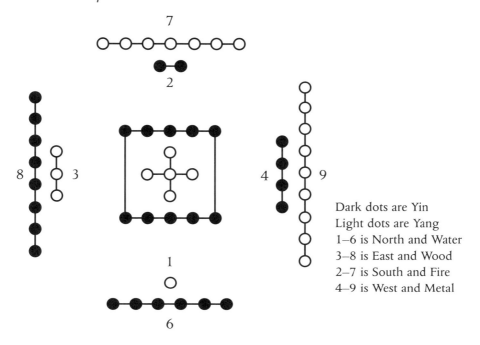

Figure 3.3 The He Tu diagram and the five phases

The He Tu pattern of the five phases is water (1–6), wood (3–8), earth (5–10), fire (2–7), and metal (4–9). The pattern begins with the number 1 and water, and follows the Yang numbers to the number 3 and wood, to the number 5 and earth, to the number 7 and fire, and to the number 9 and metal. The pattern is 1, 3, 5, 7, and 9. This is the divergent channel sequence: water is the Bladder and the Kidneys, wood is the Gallbladder and the Liver, earth is the Stomach and the Spleen, fire is the Small Intestine and the Heart, fire is also the San Jiao and the Pericardium, and metal is the Large Intestine and the Lungs. The pattern for the leg Yang channels is Bladder, Gallbladder, and Stomach; and the pattern for the leg Yin channels is Kidneys, Liver, and Spleen. The pattern for the arm Yang channels is Small Intestine, San Jiao, and Large Intestine; and that for the arm Yin channels is Heart, Pericardium, and Lungs. The He Tu has an energy pattern that contains the way channels are presented in Chapter 11 of the *Ling Shu*, "The Separate Channels." The He Tu offers supporting theory to the sequence of the divergent channels.

THE EARLY HEAVEN BA GUA

The natural school of philosophy includes Yin–Yang and the five phases theory. It is believed that these theories were developed in the Zhou dynasty (1045–221 BC), and reached a high level of sophistication in the Han dynasty (206 BC–AD 220). Most scholars and historians believe that the *Su Wen* and the *Ling Shu* were written in the Han dynasty. These books are a collection of theories and clinical experiences from many years before they were written.

The *I Ching* is considered China's oldest book, though over the centuries there were many additions to this ancient book. During the Han dynasty, Yin–Yang, five phases, and sophisticated systems of correspondences were added to it. Profound commentaries were added to the eight trigrams and the 64 hexagrams, specifically the Ten Wings. The *I Ching* includes the main philosophies of China; this ancient book includes the eight trigrams and the Ba Gua.

There are two main approaches to understanding the eight trigrams and the *I Ching*. The first method is symbolism, which includes systems of correspondences and imaging. The correspondences are models that categorize and connect all of life into Yin–Yang, five phases, the eight trigrams, the Ba Gua, and the 64 hexagrams. The second method is numbers. This approach includes the mathematical aspect of the *I Ching*. Both methods are presented to support the divergent channels pathways distribution throughout the body.

In Chinese theory there are three forces, together called San Qing. The three forces reflect universal correspondences and include the three treasures: jing, qi, and shen/heaven, humanity, and earth. The number three can mean the totality of life (and any situation). A trigram is a three-lined formation. In the *I Ching*, these three lines are combined in every possible configuration, which forms the eight trigrams. The eight trigrams have a Yin and Yang nature, and they are commonly grouped in that way. The trigrams are commonly represented in an octagon formation called a Ba Gua, which is formulated from Yin–Yang/binary theory. Figure 3.4 is the Early Heaven Ba Gua.

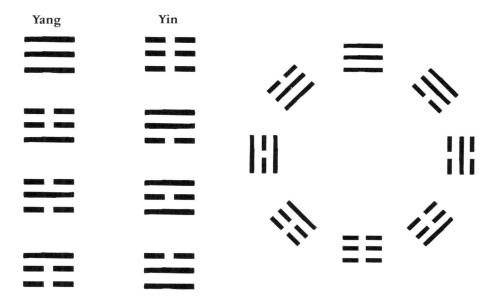

Figure 3.4 The Early Heaven Ba Gua

There are many ways to evaluate trigrams, hexagrams, and the Ba Gua. The following is an introduction to evaluating these models.

- Trigrams are evaluated from the bottom line to the top line.
- Odd numbers are Yang.
- Even numbers are Yin.
- Odd or Yang numbers consist of one stroke: ▬▬▬
- Even or Yin numbers consist of two strokes: ▬ ▬
- The number next to each trigram is the trigram position maintained in the Early Heaven Ba Gua formation—it is not the number of each trigram.

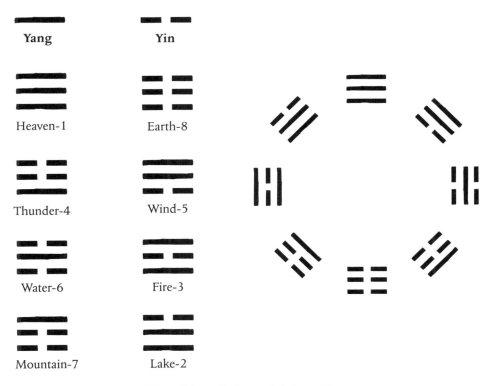

Figure 3.5 The Ba Gua and their positions

There is an inner structure of the trigrams that reflects the balanced nature of life. The following section explains important patterns that comprise this balance within the eight trigrams, the Ba Gua, and the practice of acupuncture:

- Yang trigrams contain all Yang lines, or one Yang line. Yang trigrams are Heaven, Thunder, Water, and Mountain.

- Yin trigrams contain all Yin lines, or one Yin line. Yin trigrams are Earth, Wind, Fire, and Lake.

- The total of the Yang trigrams' lines/strokes is 18.

- The total of the Yin trigrams' lines/strokes is 18.

DIVERGENT CHANNELS SEQUENCING THEORIES

- The total of the Yang trigrams' numerical positions is 1 + 4 + 6 + 7 = 18.

- The total of the Yin trigrams' numerical positions is 2 + 3 + 5 + 8 = 18.

- The sum of the strokes for each trigram set is 18. The sum of Yin and Yang trigrams is 36. Both these patterns reflect Yin–Yang balance.

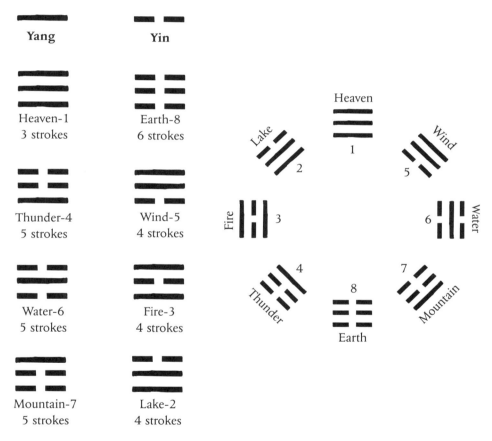

Figure 3.6 The Ba Gua and their positions and strokes

Structure of the Early Heaven Ba Gua

The Early Heaven Ba Gua is depicted in Figure 3.7. The structure of patterns within this Ba Gua embodies many forms of balance. The first analysis of the Ba Gua is to compare opposite trigrams, which includes the sum of their lines or strokes.

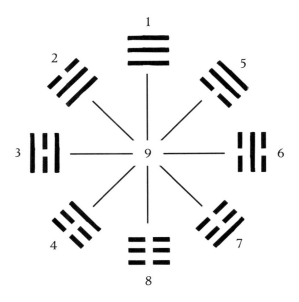

Figure 3.7 The structure of the Early Heaven Ba Gua

- The sum of the lines or strokes of Heaven-1 and Earth-8 is nine. Heaven has three strokes and Earth has six strokes.

- The sum of the lines or strokes of Mountain-7 and Lake-2 is nine. Mountain has five strokes and Lake has four strokes.

- The sum of the lines or strokes of Thunder-4 and Wind-5 is nine. Thunder has five strokes and Wind has four strokes.

- The sum of the lines of strokes of Water-6 and Fire-3 is nine. Water has five strokes and Fire has four strokes.

The second analysis of the Ba Gua shows that opposite trigrams are inverted images. For example, Heaven-1 has three Yang lines, and its opposite trigram Earth-8 has three Yin lines: they are opposite Yin–Yang polarities.

All opposite trigrams are mirror images. When there is a Yang stroke in a trigram there is a Yin stroke in the same line of its corresponding trigram. The trigrams Heaven and Earth illustrate this correspondence:

The Ba Gua contains the Yin–Yang dynamic that opposites are inverted images of polarity. Applying this inverted imaging of opposites theory to the human body reveals that corresponding areas in the body are related and can influence or treat each other.

Chapter 9 of the *Ling Shu*, "From Beginning to End," presents a treatment plan for each channel. Each treatment in this chapter includes Yin–Yang paired channels. Yin–Yang channels are considered as one inseparable channel: treating one channel influences the other channel. The channels are considered inseparable because they share the same element and are linked through internal pathways. Yin–Yang acupuncture channel pairs are presented in classic texts with little or no theory to support their relationships. The following presentation integrates multiple theories and models to support the Yin–Yang paired channels.

The Ba Gua and Yin–Yang acupuncture channel pairs

Trigrams can be organized according to their Yin and Yang quality. There are four Yin trigrams and four Yang trigrams. These trigram groupings are listed below.

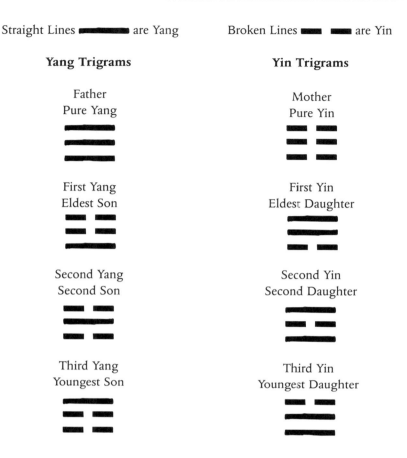

All Yang trigrams have one Yang line and two Yin lines, except Qian, which is pure Yang, and has all Yang lines. All Yin trigrams have one Yin line and two Yang lines, except Kun, which is pure Yin and contains all Yin lines. Each of the primary channels and organs is categorized according to their traditional Yin–Yang polarity. The order listed below is based on the five phases creation cycle.

Yin channels/organs are as follows:

- Wood and Liver
- Fire and Heart
- Earth and Spleen
- Metal and Lungs

- Water and Kidneys

- Wood and Pericardium.

Yang channels/organs are as follows:

- Wood and Gallbladder

- Fire and Small Intestine

- Earth and Stomach

- Metal and Large Intestine

- Water and Bladder

- Wood and San Jiao.

The acupuncture channels are matched to their corresponding trigrams based on the five phases creation cycle: wood, fire, earth, metal, and water.

Yang channels

The pattern used to assign Yang channels in this method is the five phases creation cycle and the Yin–Yang polarity of the channel.

There are four Yang trigrams. The first, Qian, contains all Yang lines; the other three have one Yang line. Based on the annual and seasonal energetics that spring and Yang wood mark the beginning of a new year and cycle, the channels are placed in the five phases creation cycle:

- Gallbladder is Yang wood and is placed with the first trigram Qian.

- Small Intestine is Yang fire and is placed with Gen.

- Stomach is Yang earth and is placed with Kan.

- Large Intestine is Yang metal and is placed with Zhen.

When those four trigrams have been matched, the pattern repeats from Qian to account for six channels matching to four trigrams. The pattern of channel placement is wood, fire, earth, metal, and water, and then repeats wood and fire to account for all six Yang channels:

Qian	Gen	Kan	Zhen
Wood	Fire	Earth	Metal
Water	Wood		
1	2	3	4
▬▬▬▬	▬▬ ▬▬	▬▬ ▬▬	▬▬ ▬▬
▬▬▬▬	▬▬▬▬	▬▬ ▬▬	▬▬ ▬▬
▬▬▬▬	▬▬ ▬▬	▬▬ ▬▬	▬▬▬▬
5	6		
GB	SI	ST	LI
BL	SJ		

The following is a step-by-step presentation of this assignment process:

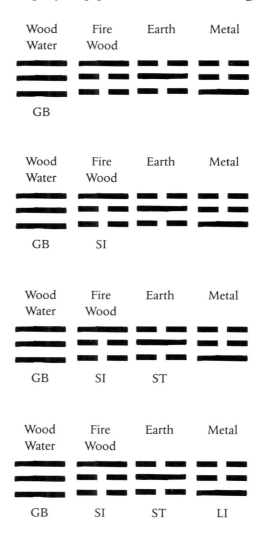

DIVERGENT CHANNELS SEQUENCING THEORIES

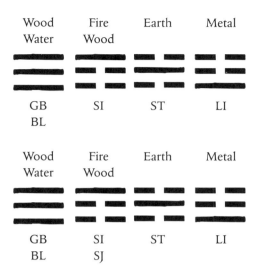

Yin channels

For Yin channels and trigrams, the same theory applies as for the Yang channels and trigrams, producing the pattern shown below:

The following is a step-by-step presentation of this assignment process:

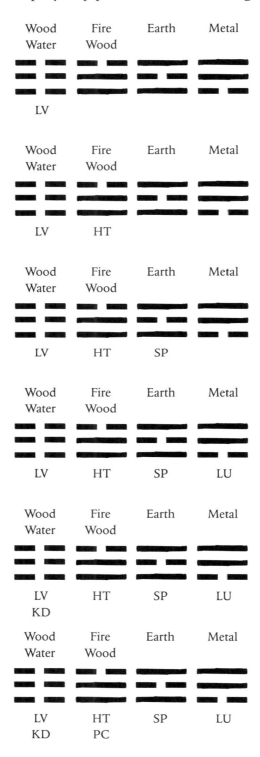

The Ba Gua and opposite channel pairs

When channel and trigram correspondences are placed on the Early Heaven Ba Gua, it shows opposite trigrams to be Yin–Yang pairs; this is Ba Gua theory supporting the Yin–Yang acupuncture channel pairings. Figure 3.8 shows these relationships. Combining Ba Gua, *Su Wen*, and *Ling Shu* theory, the Yin–Yang paired channels are revealed. Inside this Ba Gua is the exact distribution of the divergent channels on the body.

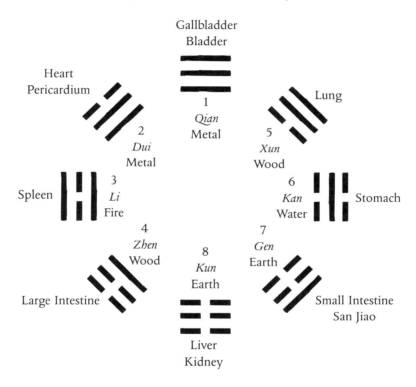

Figure 3.8 The Ba Gua and the channels

Heaven-1 and Earth-8, and Kan-6 and Li-3, represent the cardinal positions of south, north, east, and west. These trigrams and their correspondences reflect the beginning.

The four diagonal directions are Mountain-7 and Lake-2, and Thunder-4 and Wind-5. These trigrams relate to the northwest and southeast, and the northeast and southwest.

Following this pattern of trigrams reveals the following sequence of channels: Bladder and Kidneys; Gallbladder and Liver; Stomach and Spleen; Small Intestine and Heart; and Large Intestine and Lungs. The channels located at opposite trigrams are the Yin–Yang paired channels, listed in Table 3.1. When we organize this information by the Yang and Yin channels of the legs and arms, it shows the order in which the divergent channels are distributed on the body:

- The leg Yang channels are the Bladder, the Gallbladder, and the Stomach.
- The leg Yin channels are the Kidneys, the Liver, and the Spleen.
- The arm Yang channels are the Small Intestine, the San Jiao, and the Large Intestine.
- The arm Yin channels are the Heart, the Pericardium, and the Lungs.

Table 3.1 The eight trigrams and the channels

Number	Trigram	Divergent channels Yang channel sequence	Divergent channels Yin channel sequence
1	Qian–Kun Heaven–Earth 1–8	Bladder	Kidneys
2	Qian–Kun Heaven–Earth 1–8	Gallbladder	Liver
3	Kan–Li Water–Fire 3–6	Stomach	Spleen
4	Dui–Gen Lake–Mountain 2–7	Small Intestine	Heart
5	Dui–Gen Lake–Mountain 2–7	San Jiao	Pericardium
6	Zhen–Xun Thunder–Wind 4–5	Large Intestine	Lungs

When the twelve primary channels are placed into the Early Heaven Ba Gua, and Yin–Yang theory is applied to it, we find that opposite trigrams and channels confirm the sequence of the divergent channels.

The He Tu and the Early Heaven Ba Gua contain energetic distribution patterns of space that confirm the distribution of the divergent channels on the body. The He Tu and the Early Heaven Ba Gua reflect patterns of space that exist in our environment and within the human body. They are cosmic models that integrate the macrocosm and the microcosm.

CHAPTER 4

THE DIVERGENT CHANNELS

The ancient Chinese were able to perceive the inseparable nature of humanity and the universe. They developed theories and models that express and reflect this inseparable nature. Each person contains the three treasures of life: the physical, psycho-emotional, and spiritual (jing, qi, shen). These treasures are woven within the physical part of the body, including the skin, muscles, bones, organs, arteries, nerves, and the brain. They are also intertwined inside the acupuncture channels. The body and the channels are one fully integrated system. This is the insight of the ancient, natural healers.

The pathways of the acupuncture channels reflect our life. In these channels or spaces the conditions of the three treasures manifest. Because they manifest there, they can be accessed and influenced there. Depending on the healing tradition studied, a person can learn varying models for understanding the three treasures of life, and how they relate to Chinese medicine. As practitioners of three-dimensional medicine (the three treasures: jing, qi, shen/heaven, humanity, earth, etc.), we can access the channels to assist a person seeking balance. Imbalances can be found in one or more of the three dimensions of our life, and the divergent channels can access and influence the three treasures and assist in supporting a person in changing and transforming their life.

In the *Ling Shu*, there are no points listed along the pathways. As Chinese medicine developed, however, practitioners discovered areas (acupuncture points) along the pathways. These areas and points can be viewed as landmarks that can be treated. Additionally, areas along the entire pathway that have not been identified as points can and should be included in treatments. It is common in modern practice to treat one or two points on the divergent channels. However, I suggest you treat more points in order to stimulate the entire pathway. It is treating the entire pathway, not only the points listed in modern Chinese medical books, that is key to applying the divergent channels in clinical practice. A goal is to stimulate the entire channel to cause a stronger reaction in the channel, and it may take 2–8 points to do that. Each person will find the number of points and the stimulation methods that accomplish clinical results: it is a skill unique to each practitioner.

The divergent channels include junctions (confluences, unions) along their pathways. The channels have a lower and upper union. The lower junction is sometimes called earth, and the upper is called heaven. In the tables that present common points along the divergent channels, the common confluent points are listed. Some of the pathway descriptions are not precise, and more than one point may be listed as a confluent point. Examples of the confluent points are Bladder 40 and Bladder 10, the lower and upper confluent points of the Bladder and Kidney divergent channels. These two points unite both channels, and can stimulate these two divergent channels.

In this chapter, following an introduction to the fundamental qualities of the divergent channels, the channels and selected points along the pathways are presented. Learn the pathways and the points, and include both in treatments.

FUNDAMENTALS OF THE DIVERGENT CHANNELS

- The divergent channels branch out (separate) from the primary channels.

- The divergent channels flow through the major joints of the body. These are areas with large spaces. The spaces are locations where pathogens can be stored.

- The divergent channels sequence begins at the knees (Bladder–Kidneys), and then moves up to the hip, the chest, the shoulders, the throat, and the face. This is an ascending flow (the one exception is the San Jiao channel). This ascending function implies that the channels can move vital substances and pathogens upward and outward. They can also move them from the interior to the exterior. Viewing the pathways as energy fields, treating or stimulating the channels and the energy field can create an outward or inward force or reaction. The outward movement can release pathogenic factors and conditions. The inward movement can reinforce organs or maintain latency. The inward movement can draw the body's vital substances to areas or organs. By combining channel systems, the practitioner can utilize resources from the entire body to assist in a treatment. A treatment can guide the pathogen(s) through the pathways to be released, and can move pathogens up to be released by way of coughing, vomiting, sneezing, and with tears.

- Applying the classic methods of reinforcing, reducing, and dredging is an essential part of effective treatments. These needling methods send a clear message to the body about the goal and intention of the treatment, thus making treatments more effective. This is the insight and experience of the originators of acupuncture, and the tradition of the *Ling Shu*.

- The divergent channels distribute qi to the neck, face, head, and the sensory organs.

- The divergent channels flow more superficially (wei) and deeply (yuan) than the primary channels. They cover areas the primary channels do not extend into. The divergent channels also influence the middle/ying layer, due to their connections to the primary channels and the organs. The divergent channels can treat the organs. The divergent channels influence the three layers of the body: superficial, middle, and deep. They are also called the wei, ying, and yuan layers.

- The divergent channels have no points of their own. Their pathways intersect with the primary channels, and at these intersections there are acupuncture points. These points can influence both channel systems. The points with which you combine these intersection points will determine which channel or channels you are treating.

- The divergent channels can strengthen the connection of the Yin–Yang primary channels. This is the primary function presented in most texts. These channels determine six unions (confluences) of the channels and the body.

- The divergent channels connect to their associated organs. Only the divergent and primary channels connect to their organs. The divergent channels can influence the internal organs.

- The sensory organs are connected to the internal organs. Conditions of the internal organs can manifest in the sensory organs. The sensory organs are part of the elemental and the organ correspondences, which includes the five shen, and emotional and psychological conditions. Treating the sensory organs should be considered to clear the pathway of the organs, and allow the free flow of vital substances throughout the body.

These qualities listed comprise the fundamentals of the divergent channels pathways; they are essential in developing theory for clinical practice. The following section of this chapter provides you with a clear image of the pathways and acupuncture points that could be included in a treatment. As a quick reference, for each Yin–Yang channel pair there is an example of how to apply the divergent channels in clinical practice.

THE DIVERGENT CHANNELS POINTS
Bladder and Kidney
Divergent channels points

Channel	Points on the divergent channels
Bladder	Posterior of the body: Bladder 40, Bladder 36, Du 1, Bladder 32, Bladder 28, Anus, Du 4, Kidneys, Hua Tuo Jia Ji, Du 11, Bladder 15, Bladder 44, Heart, Bladder 10 Anterior of the body: Ren 3, Ren 4, Heart
Kidney	Posterior of the body: Kidney 10, Bladder 40, Du 4, Bladder 23, Bladder 52, Bladder 10 Anterior of the body: Gallbladder 26, Spleen 15, Stomach 25, Kidney 16, Ren 8 The root of the tongue loops along the jaw to Bladder 10

Confluent points

Location	Channel	Confluent point
Heaven	Kidney	Bladder 10
Earth	Bladder	Bladder 40

A Bladder and Kidney divergent channel treatment to reinforce the Kidneys could be the following:

1. Right Bladder 40
2. Right Bladder 10
3. Left Bladder 10
4. Left Bladder 40
5. Right and then left Gallbladder 26
6. Right and then left Bladder 23

These six points are on the Bladder and Kidney divergent channels.

Kidney 3 and Kidney 10 can be added to the treatment. They are the source and sea points on their respective channels.

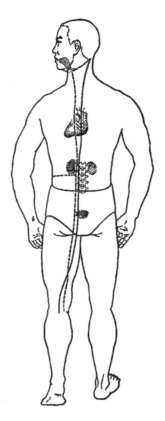

Bladder divergent channel (—)
Kidney divergent channel (---)

Gallbladder and Liver

Divergent channels points

Channel	Points on the divergent channels
Gallbladder	Gallbladder 30, Ren 2, Ren 3, Liver 13, Gallbladder 24, Gallbladder 25, Liver 14, Ren 14, Stomach 12, Ren 23, Stomach 5, Ren 24, Gallbladder 1, Liver, Heart, Throat
Liver	Liver 5, Ren 2, Gallbladder 1

Confluent points

Location	Channel	Confluent point
Heaven	Gallbladder	Gallbladder 1
Earth	Liver	Ren 2 Gallbladder 30

A Gallbladder and Liver divergent channel treatment for a male to reduce the Liver (hun imbalance) due to suppressed anger could be the following:

1. Ren 2, left Gallbladder 1, right Gallbladder 1, re-stimulate Ren 2
2. Liver 3
3. Plum blossom right Liver 5 and left Gallbladder 37

Part 1 of this treatment includes the confluent points of the channels. Reducing the points creates a vibration to release and bring to the surface (the wei layer) the imbalanced energy.

Part 2 is needling Liver 3/tai chong, the source point. This point can move qi, blood, and substances in the channel upward. When combined with the divergent channels, the flow will be upward and outward. Reinforce this point to stimulate its ability to stimulate the channels' upward and outward movement.

Part 3 includes two connecting (luo) points. They are plum blossomed, which breaks the skin and allows an outlet for the suppressed anger. In my experience, creating an outlet for the reducing method with bloodletting, plum blossom, or gua sha increases the effectiveness of the treatment.

THE DIVERGENT CHANNELS—JING BIE

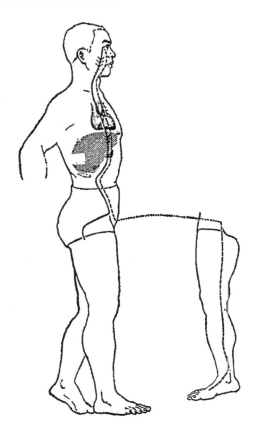

Gallbladder divergent channel (—)
Liver divergent channel (---)

Stomach and Spleen

Divergent channels points

Channel	Points on the divergent channels
Stomach	Stomach 30, Ren 12, Ren 17, Ren 22, Ren 23, Stomach 9, Stomach 4, Bladder 1
	Stomach, Spleen, Heart, Throat, and Nose
Spleen	Spleen 12, Stomach 30, Stomach 9, Ren 23, Eyes, Bladder 1

Confluent points

Location	Channel	Confluent point
Heaven	Spleen	Bladder 1
		Large Intestine 20
		Stomach 1
Earth	Stomach	Stomach 30

A Stomach and Spleen divergent channel treatment to reinforce the Spleen and Stomach could be the following:

1. Stomach 30, Large Intestine 20, Large Intestine 20, Stomach 30
2. Ren 12
3. Spleen 3, Stomach 36

The first part of the treatment includes the confluent points for the channel. I selected Large Intestine 20 because it is easier for some people to needle than Stomach 1. It is also where the Stomach primary channel begins, and it flows to Bladder 1, and then to Stomach 1. Needling Large Intestine 20 can influence all three points, and the channel circuit between them. Ren 12 is on the Stomach divergent channels pathways. It is also the mu point of the Stomach channel; it can reinforce the Stomach. Spleen 3 and Stomach 36 are the source and sea points of the Spleen and the Stomach channel. Both these points can reinforce their channels.

76 THE DIVERGENT CHANNELS—JING BIE

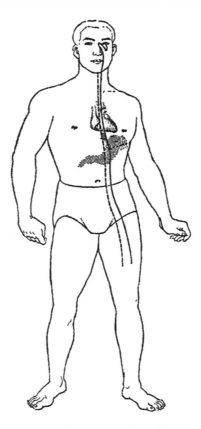

Stomach divergent channel (—)
Spleen divergent channel (---)

Small Intestine and Heart
Divergent channels points

Channel	Points on the divergent channels
Small Intestine	Small Intestine 10, Heart 1, Gallbladder 22, Ren 14, Ren 17, Stomach 12, Small Intestine 18, Bladder 1 Heart/Pericardium, Diaphragm, Small Intestine, Scapula, Throat, Root of the Tongue
Heart	Heart 1, Gallbladder 22, Ren 17, Ren 23, Bladder 1 Heart, Pericardium, Tip of the Tongue, Diffusing in the Face, the Eye

Confluent points

Location	Channel	Confluent point
Heaven	Small Intestine	Bladder 1
Earth	Heart	Gallbladder 22

A Small Intestine and Heart divergent channel treatment to reduce could be the following:

1. Gallbladder 22, Bladder 1, Small Intestine 10, Ren 14, Ren 17
2. Small Intestine 4 and 7

Gallbladder 22 and Bladder 1 are the confluent points. Treating these two points creates a vibration in the Small Intestine and Heart divergent channels. These points are reduced. The vibrational message is to release the pathogen from their divergent channels pathways and their corresponding channels.

Small Intestine 10, Ren 14, and Ren 17 are on the divergent channel pathway. Treating them assists in stimulating the pathway and releasing pathogens.

Small Intestine 4 is the source point on a Yang channel. Source points on Yang channels can assist in helping the Yang organ to empty, which is a primary function of Yang organs. Small Intestine 4 assists in releasing pathogens from the body. Small Intestine 7 is the connecting point. Perform bloodletting or plum blossom on this point to provide an outlet to more effectively release the imbalance from the body.

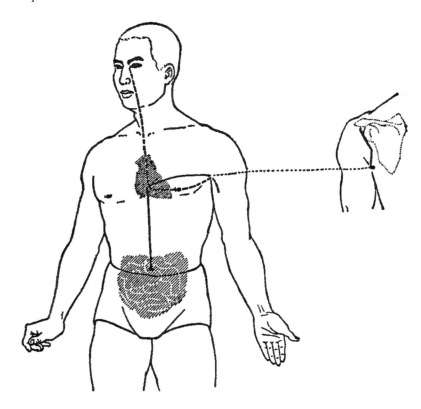

Small Intestine divergent channel (—)
Heart divergent channel (---)

San Jiao and Pericardium

Divergent channels points

Channel	Points on the divergent channels
San Jiao	Du 20, San Jiao 16, Stomach 12, Ren 17, Ren 12
	Spreads to the Chest, Pericardium
Pericardium	Pericardium 1, Ren 17, Ren 12, Ren 23, San Jiao 16
	Chest, Throat

Confluent points

Location	Channel	Confluent point
Heaven	San Jiao	San Jiao 16
		Gallbladder 12
		Small Intestine 19
Earth	Pericardium	Ren 12

A San Jiao and Pericardium divergent channel treatment to reduce could be the following:

1. Ren 12, Gallbladder 12, Ren 17, and Du 20

2. San Jiao 4 and Pericardium 8 are two of a pool of San Jiao and Pericardium channel points that could be added to the treatment.

Ren 12 and Gallbladder 12 are the confluent points on the channels. Ren 17 and Du 20 are on the divergent channels pathways. San Jiao 4 is a source point, which can help release or empty this channel (Yang channels empty). Pericardium 8 is the spring/fire point, and can clear excesses. These points would be selected for an excess condition, and for a releasing treatment.

THE DIVERGENT CHANNELS—JING BIE

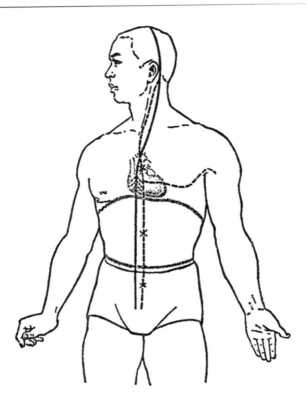

San Jiao divergent channel (—)
Pericardium divergent channel (---)

Large Intestine and Lungs

Divergent channels points

Channel	Points on the divergent channels
Large Intestine	Large Intestine 15, Du 14, Gallbladder 21, Stomach 12, Large Intestine 18, Large Intestine 15, Stomach 15 Lungs, Throat, Chest, and Breast
Lung	Lung 1, Gallbladder 22, Stomach 12, Large Intestine 18 Lungs, Breasts, Large Intestine

Confluent points

Location	Channel	Confluent point
Heaven	Large Intestine	Large Intestine 18
Earth	Lungs	Stomach 12

A Large Intestine and Lung divergent channels treatment could be the following:

1. Stomach 12, Large Intestine 18, Gallbladder 21, and Lung 1
2. Large Intestine 4

Stomach 12, Large Intestine 18, Gallbladder 21, and Lung 1 are on the divergent channels. Large Intestine 4 is the source point on a Yang channel and can help release and empty the channel and organ.

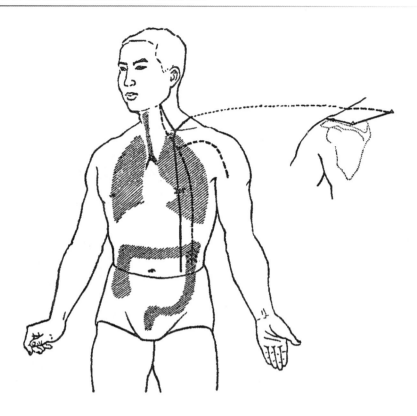

Large Intestine divergent channel (—)
Lung divergent channel (---)

THE DIVERGENT CHANNELS MAIN POINTS AND CHANNEL CONDITIONS

Table 4.1 lists the confluent and main points on the divergent channels pathways. This table is a quick reference for viewing the selected points on the channels.

Table 4.1 The divergent channels main points

Bladder	Kidney	Gallbladder	Liver
1st confluence	1st confluence	2nd confluence	2nd confluence
BL 10	BL 10	GB 1	GB 1
Heart	Along Jaw	Ren 24	Ren 2
Around Chest	Root of Tongue	ST 5	LV 5
BL 44	To the Kidney	Ren 23	
BL 15	channel	Throat	
Du 11	Ren 8	ST 12	
HTJJ (Hua Tuo Jia Ji)	KD 16	Ren 14	
Next to the Spine	SP 15	Diffuses to Heart	
Ren 4	GB 26	Liver	
Ren 3	BL 52	LV 14	
Kidneys	BL 23	GB	
Du 4	Loops around the Dai Mai	GB 24	
Anus	Du 4	GB 25	
BL 32	BL 40	LV 13	
Du 1	KD 10	Ren 3	
BL 36		Ren 2	
BL 40		GB 30	
Confluent point	Confluent point	Confluent point	Confluent point
BL 40	BL 10	GB 1	Ren 2 or GB 30

Stomach	Spleen	Small Intestine	Heart
3rd confluence	3rd confluence	4th confluence	4th confluence
BL 1	BL 1	BL 1	BL 1
Nose	Eyes	SI 18	Converge at the Eye
ST 4	Ren 23	Root of Tongue	Diffuses in Face
ST 9	Middle of the Tongue	Throat	Tip of Tongue
Ren 23	ST 9	ST 12	Ren 23
Ren 22	Throat	Scapula	Ren 17
Throat	ST 30	Ren 17	PC
Ren 17	SP 12	PC	Heart
Heart		Heart	GB 22
Diffuses into the Spleen		HT 1	HT 1
Stomach		SI 10	
Ren 12		GB 22	
ST 30		Diaphragm	
		Ren 14	
		SI	
Confluent point	Confluent point	Confluent point	Confluent point
ST 30	BL 1 or LI 20 or ST 1	BL 1	GB 22

San Jiao	Pericardium	Large Intestine	Lung
5th confluence	5th confluence	6th confluence	6th confluence
Du 20	SJ 16	Throat	LI 18
SJ 16	Ren 23	LI 18	ST 12
ST 12	Throat	Du 14	LU 1
Spreads to Chest	Ren 17	ST 12	GB 22
PC	Chest	GB 21	Lungs
Ren 17	PC 1	LI 15	Breasts
Ren 12	Ren 12	ST 15	
		Chest	
		Breast	
		Diffuses to Lungs	
		LI	
Confluent point	Confluent point	Confluent point	Confluent point
SJ 16 or GB 12, SJ 19	Ren 12	St 12	LI 18

ROOTS AND ENDS

Chapter 5 of the *Ling Shu* presents "Roots and Ends," describing the link between the internal organs and the divergent channels. It describes a specific root (beginning) and end of the channels. Some of the beginnings and endings are different than the common union (confluent) points. According to the *Ling Shu*: "it is at these beginnings and endings that pathogens from the primary channels and organs can enter the divergent channels." Consider using these points in clinical practice, especially when the condition includes these regions.

In the "Roots and Ends" chapter, it is said:

> For one who comprehends ends and beginnings, one sentence is enough. For one who does not understand ends and beginnings, the way of the needle is completely cut off.[9]

The roots and ends are locations to treat. Table 4.2 presents these points.

Table 4.2 Roots and ends

Channel	Root begins	Ending ends	Anatomical area of the ending
Tai Yang	Bladder 67	Bladder 1	Eyes
Shao Yang	Gallbladder 44	Small Intestine 19	Ear
Yang Ming	Stomach 45	Stomach 8	Corner of the Head
Tai Yin	Spleen 1	Ren 12	Stomach
Shao Yin	Kidney 1	Ren 23	Throat
Jue Yin	Liver 1	Ren 17	Chest

Consider treating the beginnings and endings in treatments, along with the confluent and pathway points. The confluent or root and end points can be used to begin a divergent channel treatment. The root and end points begin on the extremities, located in areas where there are no confluent points. Thus they offer additional ways to treat the divergent channels. Confluent and root and end points can stimulate the pathways and begin the process of reinforcing and reducing. They send a message to the channel system that is being treated. The key to effective treatments is developing the ability to find the right amount of additional points for an effective treatment.

Part II
WORKING IT OUT

CHAPTER 5

THE MAJOR AND CONNECTING CHANNELS

> The major channels make the beginning. They manage and nourish the substances that flow throughout the body. They create the depths and limits of the body. Internally, they connect to the five Yin organs. Externally, they are distributed to the six Yang organs.
>
> The major channels can decide life and death. They are the locations of the hundred diseases. They also can harmonize emptiness and fullness. This cannot be done if they are not understood.[10]

The major channels of acupuncture (the primary channels) are the main channels treated in modern acupuncture. These channels are presented in the *Ling Shu*, Chapter 10, "The Major Channels"; it is the fundamental chapter on the primary channels and presents each of the twelve channel pathways, as well as the pathogens, conditions, and diseases that occur when the channels suffer from excess, deficiency, and stagnations. The chapter includes conditions of the channels, as well as conditions of the internal organs. In most Chinese medical schools the internal organ (the zang fu) energetics are emphasized; however, often the channel energetics are not emphasized.

There are two main ways to view conditions of the channels. The first are the signs and symptoms found in the *Ling Shu*, "The Major Channels." The second way is when there are conditions along the pathway of the channel. It is common when treating pain to identify the channel affected, and then treat that channel. For some practitioners, treating the conditions along a channel, and the set of symptoms presented in this Chapter 10, may be new. Chapters 5, 9, and 10 of the *Ling Shu* present the physiology and pathology of the channels, providing the foundation for clinical practice.

This chapter lists the major conditions found in "The Major Channels." When these conditions exist, treat the primary channels. Also consider treating their associated divergent channels to support the treatment goal of reducing, reinforcing, or dredging.

THE MAJOR CHANNELS

The Hand Tai Yin channel
The Lung channel

Conditions include coughing, rebellious qi, panting and thirst, an anxious Heart, a congested chest, pain and spasms in the shoulder bone and the medial anterior surface of the upper arm, and heat in the center of the palm. When the qi is full and there is excess, it results in the shoulder and back being painful from wind and cold. There will be sweating from the attacking wind. Urination is frequent but scanty. When qi is empty, it results in the shoulder and back being painful from cold. Sparse qi is in accord with an insufficiency of breathing. There will be change in the color of urine.

The Hand Yang Ming channel
The Large Intestine channel

There are toothaches and swelling of the neck. This channel transports the body fluids, and may be the source of diseases where the symptoms are yellow eyes, a dry mouth, a runny nose, nosebleed, sore throat, pain in the anterior part of the shoulder or upper arm, and pain and nonfunctioning of the thumb and index finger. When the qi is in excess, the areas the channel passes through are hot and swollen. When the qi is empty, the result is cold, chills, and poor circulation.

The Foot Yang Ming channel
The Stomach channel

Diseases include shaking from cold as if one is sprinkled with water, frequent groaning, frequent yawning, and the forehead is black. A disease state causes the person to feel sick from fire, and to be timid and fearful when hearing tones are resonant to wood. While the Heart desires motion, one stays alone behind blocked doors and closed shutters. In extremes, it results in the desire to ascend heights and sing and cast off one's clothes while walking outside. There are noises in the abdomen, and swelling caused by a deficiency around the shinbone. This channel controls the blood and the diseases which arise from it: madness, fevers, warm diseases, debauchery, abnormal sweating, bleeding from the nose, a dry mouth, canker of the lips, swelling of the neck, numbness in the throat, water retention in the abdomen, and swelling and pain in the knee and knee cap. There is also pain along the shoulder and breast, qi rushing, pain in the abdomen, the thighs, the front of the thigh, the lateral side of the leg bone, the upper part of the foot and ankle, and the middle toe does not function. When the qi is in excess, it results in the front of the body being hot. So when there is an excess of qi in the Stomach, it results in a melting of grains, frequent hunger, and yellow-colored urine. When the qi is insufficient, it causes the front of the body to shiver with cold. When the middle of the Stomach is cold, it results in swelling and fullness.

The Foot Tai Yin channel
The Spleen channel

The root of the tongue is rigid, there can be vomiting after eating, and there is pain in the ducts of the Stomach, swelling of the abdomen, frequent regurgitation, a gaseous discharge after a bowel movement, and body heaviness. The channel controls the Spleen and gives rise to disease where the root of the tongue is painful, the body is unable to move or swing, and food does not descend. There is anxiety in the Heart, acute pain below the Heart, watery stools, blocked water, yellow jaundice, an inability to lie down, rigidity in standing, swelling and deficiency of the interior of the thighs and knees, and the big toes do not function.

The Hand Shao Yin channel
The Heart channel

There is a dry throat and the Heart is painful. There is a deficiency of the upper arm. There can be yellow eyes, the ribs hurt, and the medial posterior surface of the upper arm is cold and painful. The center of the palm is hot and painful.

The Hand Tai Yang channel
The Small Intestine channel

There can be a sore throat, the chin and jaws are swollen, the neck is stiff and immobile, the shoulder feels as if it is pulled apart, and the upper part of the arm feels as if it is broken. There may be deafness, yellow eyes, swollen cheeks, and pain in the neck, jaws, shoulder, upper arm, elbow, and the lateral posterior side of the arm.

The Foot Tai Yang channel
The Bladder channel

There can be rushes to the head, painful eyes, the nape of the neck feels tight and constrained, the spine is painful, the loins feel as if they are broken, the hips are unable to bend, the knee feels tied up, and the calf feels as if it were separated. There is a deficiency of qi at the ankle. *This channel controls the tendons* and gives rise to diseases such as piles, fevers, madness and insanity, pain in the top of the head and in the nape of the neck, yellow eyes, tearing, and nosebleeds. There can be pain in the back, loins, buttocks, knees, calves, and the feet. The little toe does not function.

The Foot Shao Yin channel
The Kidney channel

One may feel hungry but does not desire to eat, the face is black like charcoal, there is blood from coughing or spitting, and there is a desire to arise when sitting. The eyes are blurred so that they are without perception. When the qi is insufficient, it results in fear. The Heart is frightened and distressed.

This is a deficiency in the bones. This channel controls the Kidneys and gives rise to diseases where there is fever in the mouth, a dry tongue, a swollen throat, an upward flow of qi, the throat dry and sore, anxiety in the Heart, pain in the Heart, jaundice, diarrhea, pain in the spine, flaccidity, a fondness for lying down, and the bottom of the foot is hot and painful.

The Hand Jue Yin channel
The Pericardium channel

The palms of the hand may feel hot, the forearm and elbow being distorted and stiff, and there may be swelling in the armpit. In extreme cases there is fullness in the chest and ribs, and palpitations of the Heart. The face can become red and the eyes may become a yellow color. There can be persistent laughter. This channel controls the blood channels and pulse, and may give rise to anxiety.

The Hand Shao Yang channel
The San Jiao channel

Conditions can include deafness and tinnitus. There can be swelling and a sore throat. This channel controls the qi and may give rise to diseases where there is abnormal sweating. There can be pain at the lateral corner of the eye, at the cheek or jaw behind the ear, and in the shoulder and the upper limb. There can be a dysfunction of the ring finger.

The Foot Shao Yang channel
The Gallbladder channel

There can be a bitter taste in the mouth and frequent belching. There can be pain in the Heart and ribs, and the inability to turn or to lean. When extreme, it results in the face looking slightly ashen, the body being without oil and dry, and the lateral side of the foot being hot. This is from the Yang being deficient. *This channel controls the bones* and can cause diseases such as headache, and pain in the chin, jaw, and lateral corner of the eyes. There can be swelling and pain in the center of the Broken Dish, swelling below the armpits, goiters under the arms, abnormal sweating caused by chills and fevers, and pains in the breast, ribs, buttocks, and knees along the lateral surface of the fibula bone to the lower end and the area in front of the lateral malleolus and all the joints. The fourth toe may not function properly.

The Foot Jue Yin channel
The Liver channel

There can be pain in the groin area, and one may not be able to bend down or look up. There can be hernias in men, and abdominal swellings in women. In extreme cases there can be a dry throat, an ashen face, and a pale complexion. *This channel controls the Liver* and may give rise to diseases such as fullness of the breast, vomiting, hiccups, diarrhea, recurrent hernia, and weak or blocked urine.

In modern applications of traditional Chinese medicine (TCM) the internal organs often take priority in diagnosis and treatment. The predominant diagnostic and treatment model is zang fu. In classical acupuncture, the internal organs are one aspect of the body that is evaluated to make a diagnosis and treatment plan. Pathogens and imbalances can be located in the channels (not the organs) and throughout the body. Imbalances of the organs can be transferred into the divergent channels pathways. In either case, the divergent channels can be used to treat pathogens in the divergent channels pathways, as well as supporting the primary channel's ability to treat an organ condition.

CONDITIONS OF THE INTERNAL ORGANS

A simplified list of the standard conditions related to the internal organs is now presented. When these appear and an organ diagnosis is made, consider using the corresponding divergent channel in a treatment.

The Lungs

Cough, asthma, shortness of breath, sputum, hemoptysis, weak voice, fatigue, frequent colds, chest pain with a stifling sensation, palpitations, restlessness, unsmooth frequent urination, incontinence, edema, abdominal fullness/distension, loose stools, diarrhea, constipation, and burning pain in the epigastrium or behind the sternum.

The Large Intestine

Abdominal pain, pain around umbilicus, borborygmus, flatulence, sticky diarrhea, constipation, cough, asthma, sputum, chest pain, low energy, epigastric pain, vomiting, belching, facial edema, sweating or lack of sweating, and thirst.

The Stomach

Yangming fu conditions, tidal fever, constipation, focal distension/fullness in the abdomen, frequent hunger, feeling of emptiness in the Stomach, indigestion, distension/pain in the epigastrium/abdomen, nausea, vomiting, diarrhea, constipation, borborygmus, ascites, manic depression, abnormal mental function, and abnormal yawning (moaning).

The Spleen

Epigastric pain, loose stools, diarrhea, borborygmus, vomiting, nausea, abdominal fullness/distension, reduced appetite, jaundice, lassitude, listlessness, abdominal qi masses, leucorrhea, excess phlegm fluid, difficult urination, and edema.

The Heart

Cardiac pain, palpitations, irregular Heart beat, shortness of breath, restlessness, mental abnormality, insomnia, dream-disturbed sleep, sudden fainting, hysteria, shallow breathing, esophagitis, and hiatal hernia.

The Small Intestine

Yellow urination, urinary retention, edema, diarrhea, constipation, Stomach/abdominal pain, distending qi pain in the lower abdomen relating to the lumbar area and testicles, and inguinal hernia.

The urinary Bladder
Unsmooth urination with distension and pain in the lower abdomen, urinary retention, enuresis, dysmenorrhea, leucorrhea, manic depression, epilepsy, excess worry, phobia, fears, opisthotonos, and malaria.

The Kidneys
Facial puffiness, edema, impotence, infertility, forgetfulness, dizziness, blurred vision, dark circles under eyes, dark/withered complexion, dark spots on skin, loose stools, chronic diarrhea or constipation, abdominal distension, hunger with no desire to eat, vomiting, nausea, restlessness, insomnia or somnolence, palpitations, cardiac pain, anxiety, sensation of qi rushing upward to chest/head, shortness of breath, labored breathing, chronic cough, easily fatigued, and fear, anxiety, and being easily frightened causing palpitations.

The Pericardium
Palpitations, cardiac pain, restlessness, stuffiness in chest, delirium, syncope, incessant laughing, depression, anxiety, and manic depression.

The San Jiao
Puffiness, edema, enuresis, urinary retention, frequent urination, chest pain, cough, palpitations, epigastric pain, vomiting, nausea, abdominal distension/fullness, constipation, diarrhea, hypothyroidism, hyperthyroidism, diabetes, and tumors/masses/fibroids/cysts.

The Gallbladder
Hypochondriac pain, vomiting, nausea, belching, bitter taste in mouth, poor appetite, abnormal bowel movements, dusky/dark complexion, swelling/pain in scrotum, hernia, leucorrhea, itching/pain at the external genitalia, difficult urination, deep sighing, depression, mood swings, frequent anger, poor judgment, indecision, and insomnia.

The Liver

Hypochondriac pain/fullness/distension, dizziness, blurred vision, tinnitus, dry throat, flushed face, fever, jaundice, bitter taste, nervousness, depression, mood swings, frequent anger, frustration, epigastric distension, belching, flatulence, eating disorders, nausea, vomiting, abdominal pain/distension, irregular menstruation, infertility, impotence, itching external genitalia, leucorrhea, epididymitis, enuresis, urinary retention, yellow urine, stuffiness of chest, cough with blood in the sputum, shallow breathing, deep sighing, palpitations, dream-disturbed sleep, abnormal growths (masses/nodules/fibroids/cysts), and plum pit syndrome.

THE CONNECTING CHANNELS (THE LUO CHANNELS)

The connecting channels are presented in Chapter 10 of the *Ling Shu*, "The Major Channels." This chapter presents the pathways and imbalances of the primary channels, as well as the connecting (luo) channels. We can assume that because the primary and the connecting channels are presented in the same chapter they have a direct relationship with each other. The imbalances in each of the channels can transfer between each other. This relationship is an example of the interrelated nature of the channel system.

A unique insight of the early Chinese practitioners is that emotions are stored in the blood, and the connecting channels treat blood. Consequently, they can treat emotions. And the channels that influence the connecting and primary channels can also assist in treating emotions; they are the divergent channels.

"The Major Channels" presents the connecting (luo) points and the connecting channels pathology. Table 5.1 summarizes the connecting channel pathology from that chapter.

Table 5.1 The connecting channel pathology

Channel	Excess pathology	Deficient pathology
Lung	Heat in the wrist and palm	Yawning and frequent urination
Heart	Fullness and pressure in the chest and diaphragm	Loss of speech
Pericardium	Heart pain	Vexation in the Heart
Large Intestine	Toothache, deafness	Teeth sensitive to cold, bi conditions
Small Intestine	Loosening of the joints and lack of muscle tone of the sinews in the elbow area	Small swellings
San Jiao	Spasms and cramps of the muscles around the elbow	Lack of muscle tone of the elbows
Stomach	Counterflow qi in the channel, throat bi, and sudden loss of voice	Lack of muscle tone of the feet and a withering of the shins
Bladder	Nasal congestion with clear nasal discharge, headache, back pain	Clear nasal discharge, bloody nose
Gallbladder	Inversion	Weakness and lack of muscle tone of the lower limbs with inability to stand from a sitting position
Spleen	Cholera, stabbing pain in the intestines	Drum-like distension of the abdomen
Kidney	Vexation and oppression, constipation and urinary block	Lower back pain
Liver	Swelling in the testicles, abnormal erection	Sudden genital itching
Ren	Pain in the skin of the abdomen	Itching in the skin of the abdomen
Du	Rigidity of the back	Sensation of heaviness of the head, shaking the head
Great luo of Spleen	Aching and pain of the whole body	Looseness of the hundred joints

In his book *Guide to Acupuncture* (1196),[11] Dou Han Qing presented a method of using source and luo points of the Yin–Yang paired channels. He used what would become known as the transverse connecting channels (transverse luo channels), and an application of the guest and host acupuncture treatment. It appears there is no reference to these channels (transverse channel branches) in classical Chinese texts. For this reason, some practitioners do not use this method. The classics suggest using the Yin–Yang paired channels in treatments; they do not designate the source and luo points as a way to more effectively treat the channels. They make no reference of *transverse* channels. According to this theory, it is these transverse channels that allow a transfer of qi from one of the channels to the other. This idea would become a common method used in the future. Dou Han Qing was also the person that revealed the eight master (opening, confluent) points of the eight extraordinary channels.

The primary channels, the internal organs, and the connecting channels are associated with unique diseases, conditions, signs, and symptoms. Because the divergent channels are connected to each of these channels and organs, they can assist in treating them. Yin–Yang theory contains the principle that combining two or more channels can cause a stronger reaction and effect in the body than treating one channel. The divergent channels are a potent channel system to support the primary and connecting channels presented in this chapter, as well as the internal organs. Using these channels in treatments is applying Yin–Yang theory in clinical practice.

CHAPTER 6

CYCLES OF TIME

> On understanding the moving power and its way: the onset of a therapeutic effect is faster than shooting an arrow. Without understanding the moving power and the Dao, effects are wasted, like arrows failing to leave the bow. To understand their comings and goings, emphasize the appropriate cycle of times. Ordinary doctors are in the dark; wondrous are the few who possess the unique skills.[12]

Time and space are essential aspects of Chinese medicine. Space is the body, which includes the organs and the acupuncture channels. Time is cycles of time. These cycles include the nourishing qi cycle (daily clock), the muscle channels cycles, the wei qi cycle, and the yearly, seasonal, and monthly cycles. Pathogens can flow with cycles of time and be transferred throughout the body (space) during the cycles. Time and space are inseparable. This chapter presents important cycles of time and their relationships to the spaces in the body.

THE NOURISHING QI CYCLE

The *Ling Shu*, Chapter 16, "The Nourishing Qi," presents the cycle of nourishing qi (ying qi). This cycle is also known as the daily or meridian clock (see Figure 6.1). The chapter assigns no times to the channels and their sequence. It presents the standard sequence of the channels found in Chinese medical books. It describes a very important sequence in the cycle that is not commonly presented.

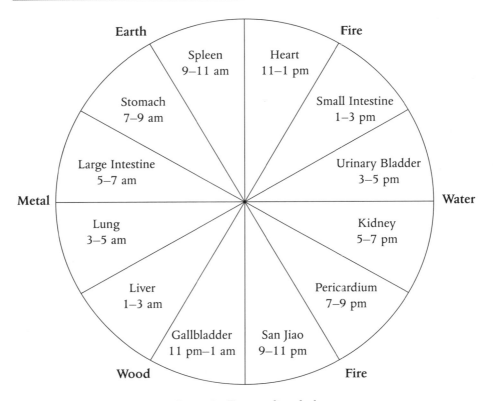

Figure 6.1 The meridian clock

All presentations begin with the nourishing qi originating in the Stomach, which then flows to the Lungs, Large Intestine, Stomach, Spleen, Heart, Small Intestine, Bladder, Kidneys, Pericardium, San Jiao, Gallbladder, and Liver. All presentations state that the cycle flows from the Liver back to the Lungs. The *Ling Shu* states that the cycle flows from the Liver to the Lungs, and then a branch flows to the throat, the nasal passages, the forehead, the top of the head, and down to the nape of the neck and spine to the coccyx; this is the *Du channel*. It then flows up the front of the body to the navel and abdomen, to Stomach 12/Broken Dish, and then descends to the Lung channel. This flow up the front of the body is the *Ren channel*.

The nourishing cycle includes post-natal substances from the food and fluid we digest and process. That is on the physical dimension. It also includes the psycho-emotional dimension related to the five shen and the five Yin organs. The portion of the nourishing qi cycle that flows to the Du and Ren channels is a path for post-natal influences, the emotions, to move to the deep (yuan) levels in the body. In other words, emotions and experiences that are not resolved will enter into the eight extraordinary channels, and can potentially become part of our constitution.

The perpetual flow of this cycle can nourish and rejuvenate the organs, channels, and the entire body with ying qi. This cycle can also circulate pathogens and unfavorable emotions throughout the body. If the condition is not resolved, it will go into the organs and influence their physical function, as well as the psycho-emotional and spiritual condition. The five shen can be influenced because they are housed in the organs.

Understanding the way that this cycle flows provides a guide to treating conditions. When lifestyle creates imbalances, they can flow from the post-natal level to the deep yuan level. The ying qi cycle illustrates this possibility and is a reminder to resolve minor post-natal conditions before they become more severe.

The nourishing qi cycle contains time and space; it is a cycle of heaven and earth. Time is heaven and space is earth. Space is the channels, organs, and locations the cycle circulates throughout the body. This flow occurs throughout our lifetime. Time is the daily clock aspect. In the long history of Chinese medicine, the time of the day and its influence on the body was identified and studied. This insight led to the daily clock. When a condition occurs during specific times it may indicate that organ and channel are part of a health condition. Symptoms at this time should lead the practitioner to evaluate that channel and organ system. Table 6.3 later in the chapter lists the twelve organs and channels, and their corresponding times.

Imbalances in the primary channels and the internal organs can be driven deeper into the body by the perpetual circulation of the nourishing qi cycle. These conditions can also be moved or transferred to other channels, including the divergent channels. The clinical applications of the divergent channels include clearing pathogens from their own channels, as well as providing the energy or an energetic force to assist the primary channels to release the pathogens in their organs or channels. This relationship, which shows the inter-relationship of the acupuncture channel system and the human body, is essential in the practice of acupuncture. Including this understanding in clinical practice will allow the practitioner to utilize numerous aspects of the body to treat a condition. There is a potent synergy that occurs when the multiple aspects of the body are unified in a single treatment plan.

THE MUSCLE CHANNELS AND BONES

The *Ling Shu*, Chapter 13, "The Muscle Channels," describes the muscle channels and their diseases. The muscle channels are also called the sinew or tendon-muscle channels. These channels are large regions that include tendons, muscles, and the skeleton system. The chapter presents diseases of each of the twelve muscle channels, and also describes a unique aspect of time and space, which is the relationship between the channels and the months of the year. Each channel relates to one month, and each channel is more susceptible to disease in its corresponding month. Table 6.1 presents the muscle channels and the months of the year.

Table 6.1 The muscle channels and the twelve lunar months

Month	Muscle channel
January	Gallbladder
February	Bladder
March	Stomach
April	Large Intestine
May	Small Intestine
June	San Jiao
July	Kidney
August	Spleen
September	Liver
October	Pericardium
November	Lung
December	Heart

When a condition consistently occurs or is aggravated during a specific month, consider the related organ and channel system for evaluation, diagnosis, and treatment. Consider treating a channel during its month; this is a variation of treating a channel during its two-hour daily cycle.

WEI QI CIRCULATION

Ying qi and wei qi are post-natal substances. These two substances flow throughout the body based on a daily cycle. The ying qi flows in the acupuncture channels, and wei qi flows at the superficial layers of the body: in the muscle channels (muscles, tendons, or sinew channels). The circulation begins when awakening and opening the eyes. Opening the eyes begins a pattern of two hours for the wei qi flow in each muscle channel. Table 6.2 presents the twelve double-hour pattern.

Table 6.2 The wei qi and the muscle channels cycle

Channel	Muscle channel	Organ name	Begins when awakening
3-Leg Yang	Tai Yang	Bladder	2 hours
	Shao Yang	Gallbladder	2 hours
	Yang Ming	Stomach	2 hours
3-Arm Yang	Tai Yang	Small Intestine	2 hours
	Shao Yang	San Jiao	2 hours
	Yang Ming	Large Intestine	2 hours
3-Leg Yin	Tai Yin	Spleen	2 hours
	Shao Yin	Kidney	2 hours
	Jue Yin	Liver	2 hours
3-Arm Yin	Tai Yin	Lung	2 hours
	Shao Yin	Heart	2 hours
	Jue Yin	Pericardium	2 hours

The wei qi cycle can be used as a diagnostic tool. If a person's condition of the muscle channels appears or intensifies during a certain time of the day, note the muscle channel for that time of the day. The time and its channel can lead the practitioner to identify a specific channel for further examination.

The divergent channels can assist in releasing pathogens in the muscle channels. Because the divergent channels are part of a network of channels, they can provide the qi or force to assist in releasing the pathogens; for example, heat, cold, wind, or dampness. And they can release pathogens that have transferred from the muscle channels to the divergent channels. This release would include treating the divergent channels to move the pathogen outward, and then a muscle channel treatment to release it from the body.

MAIN CONDITIONS OF THE MUSCLE CHANNELS

The main conditions of the muscle channels are listed in the *Ling Shu*, Chapter 13, "The Muscle Channels." The conditions are now listed here.

The Foot Tai Yang channel
The Bladder channel

Conditions include swelling and pain in the little toe and heel. Spasms can occur at the crease of the knee and the neck muscles. Cramps and pain can occur in the pathway from the armpit to the center of Broken Dish (Stomach 12). There can be an inability to raise the shoulders. And there can be a backward-bent backbone.

The Foot Shao Yang channel
The Gallbladder channel

Conditions include muscle spasms of the fourth toe, the lateral side of the knee, and the crease of the knee, ranging to the thigh and buttocks. The spasms can lead to the inability to bend or stretch. There can be pain in the ribs, which can range to Broken Dish (Stomach 12) and the neck. The eyes cannot open if the spasms move from the left to the right, and from the right to the left. The left and right are interconnected, and they influence each other. This is the mutual intercourse of connected muscles.

The Foot Yang Ming channel
The Stomach channel

Conditions include muscle spasms of the middle toe, the leg, and the Crouching Rabbit (Stomach 32). There can be swelling on the front of the thigh. There can be a hernia, and spasms ranging from the abdomen to Broken Dish, and the cheek. The mouth may spasm. The eyes may not be able to close. If there is heat, the muscles may relax and the eyes may not open. If the muscles of the cheek are cold, it causes spasms and will induce twisting of the cheek and the mouth. If there is heat, it will cause the muscles to relax deeply; this makes the muscle unable to contract and causes a distortion.

The Foot Tai Yin channel
The Spleen channel

Conditions can include pain in the big toe and the medial ankle. There may be pain and spasms of the muscles along the leg bone, and the medial side of the knees and thigh where the pathway leads to the upper thigh. There can be knotting pain in the sexual organs, which can lead up to the navel and both flanks, and cause pain in the chest and the center of the spine.

The Foot Minor Yin channel
The Kidney channel

Conditions include muscle spasms in the bottom of the foot. Conditions also include epilepsy, spasms, and cramps. When the back is affected, one cannot bend forward. When the front is affected, one cannot bend backward.

The Foot Jue Yin channel
The Liver channel

Conditions include pain in the big toe and along the channel up to the front of the medial ankle, the medial side of the leg, and pain and spasms in the muscles at the inner thigh. Injury to these muscles and channels can influence the sexual organs and result in the inability to maintain an erection. Cold can cause contractions of the sexual organs. Heat causing injury can result in an abnormally long erection.

The Hand Tai Yang channel
The Small Intestine channel

Conditions can include pain in the little finger along the pathway to the elbow on the medial side, and behind the medial epicondyle, as well as pain along the Yin side of the upper arm, the area below the armpit, the bottom of the armpit, and on the surface behind the armpit, and pain which winds around the shoulder blade, which in turn includes pain in the neck. There are correspondences between ringing in the middle of the ear and pain in the chin and jaws, delayed vision after prolonged closing of the eyes, and spasms in the neck muscles, which can cause ulcers and swellings in the neck, and chills and heat at the neck.

The Hand Shao Yang channel
The San Jiao channel

Conditions include cramps of the muscles at the points that flow along the pathway. The spasms can cause a rolled-up tongue.

The Hand Yang Ming channel
The Large Intestine channel

Conditions include cramping of the muscles at the areas along the pathways. There can be an inability to raise the shoulder or to turn the neck to the left or right.

The Hand Tai Yin channel
The Lung channel

Conditions include cramping of the muscles along its pathways. Extreme pain in the cardiac orifice may cause panting. Spasms in the ribs may cause the spitting of blood.

The Hand Shao Yin channel
The Heart channel

Conditions include spasms of the Heart. They may make the elbow feel as if it is in a net. The diseases of this muscle channel include pain and cramping along its pathway.

The Hand Jue Yin channel
The Pericardium channel

Conditions include cramping of the muscles along the pathways, including the sternum, and the cardiac area.

MEASUREMENTS IN REFERENCE TO THE BONES

The *Ling Shu*, Chapter 14, "Measurements in Reference to the Bones," presents information about bones. The chapter describes the length of the major bones of the body. In Chinese medicine, jing (essence and source qi) is in the bones. In Western medicine, stem cells are in the bones. The bones contain some of the most powerful substances in the body. Influencing bones with acupuncture, herbs, or exercise influences the substances in the bones.

Because the muscle channels connect to bones, they can influence jing and source qi. From an anatomical layer perspective, bones are at the superficial layer (they connect to tendons and muscles), which is the wei layer. From the vital substance layer perspective, bones are part of the yuan or deep level. Bones are part of the marrow matrix and are connected to the eight extraordinary channels, jing, and source qi. Bones are a medium of the superficial (wei) and deep (yuan) layers, which include the defensive and source qi. The divergent channels flow from the exterior to the interior, from the wei to the yuan layers. The divergent channels influence both layers. They can release conditions from the deep layers to the superficial layers, assisting in releasing them out of the body. The divergent channels can also guide the body's substances from the wei layer to the yuan layer.

This movement from the superficial to the deep areas of the body is commonly used to reinforce. It can also be used to maintain a condition until a person is ready to deal with the condition. It can maintain latency.

The large bones have muscles and spaces (joints) surrounding them. Pathogens can accumulate in these locations. If they are not cleared they can create chronic health conditions. Divergent channel treatments have a potent influence on bones and the spaces near them. This is the space aspect of time and space.

The confluent points of the divergent channels are mostly located at a bone structure. From these bone structures the pathways flow throughout the body. Having clarity of the relationships of bones and these channels is essential in understanding the clinical applications of the divergent channels. The condition of bones is vital in Western and Chinese medicine. The skeletal system is a link between the anatomical structures of the body, as well as the vital substances (wei qi and yuan qi). It is also a protective structure to major internal organs. The divergent channels generally begin and end at bones, and they can influence bones and their associated anatomical structures, vital substances, pathogens, and acupuncture channels. These relationships are a reason why divergent channels can support all the channels.

CHINESE MEDICAL ASTROLOGY

Chinese medical astrology is a traditional way to understand a person and the cycles of time in their life. One simple application is to use the hour of birth. Based on the daily clock, each two-hour time frame relates to a channel and organ. Table 6.3 contains the double hours and the related channel and organ.

Table 6.3 The hour stem and branch table

Time	Organ	Source point
11 pm–1 am	Gallbladder	Gallbladder 40
1 am–3 am	Liver	Liver 3
3 am–5 am	Lung	Lung 9
5 am–7 am	Large Intestine	Large Intestine 4
7 am–9 am	Stomach	Stomach 42
9 am–11 am	Spleen	Spleen 3
11 am–1 pm	Heart	Heart 7
1 pm–3 pm	Small Intestine	Small Intestine 4
3 pm–5 pm	Bladder	Bladder 64
5 pm–7 pm	Kidney	Kidney 3
7 pm–9 pm	Pericardium	Pericardium 7
9 pm–11 pm	San Jiao	San Jiao 4

Locate the hour of birth in the hour stem and branch table, and then identify the organ for the hour of birth. A person is susceptible to conditions related to their hour of birth's corresponding organ. For example, a person born between 5 pm and 7 pm is susceptible to Kidney conditions. As a preventative practice, press or massage the source point of the organ of your hour of birth each day. For 5 pm to 7 pm, it is Kidney 3.

The nourishing qi cycle, the wei qi cycle, the muscle channel cycle, and the Chinese medical astrology cycle are all cycles of time. These cycles can be included in making a diagnosis.

CHAPTER 7

THE FIVE SHEN

> In the human body there are the five yin (zang) internal organs of the Heart, Spleen, Lungs, Kidneys, and the Liver. The organs provide the structure and the qi to form and allow the manifestation of the five spirits, which then gives rise to the five natural virtues and emotions.[13]

The ancient Chinese observed their environment and noticed the effects of nature on their body, mind, and spirit (the three treasures). The relationship between the environment and the three treasures of each person comprises an essential aspect of the Chinese healing arts. A profound insight of the Chinese healers was the inseparable relationship between the body and the psycho-emotional condition. The psychological condition influences the body, and the body influences the psychological condition. These ancient healers developed ways to express the relationship between the body and the mind. One way of expressing the relationship of the body, mind, and spirit is the *Su Wen* and *Ling Shu* model of the five shen. The five shen can be interpreted as five aspects of the consciousness and personality. The five shen is an effective model for making a diagnosis and developing a treatment plan for treating emotional, psychological, and spiritual conditions.

The five shen are presented in the *Su Wen*, Chapter 5, "The Manifestation of Yin and Yang from the Macrocosm to the Microcosm," and in the *Ling Shu*, Chapter 8, "Roots and Spirit." Chapter 5 of the *Su Wen* presents the relationship between nature, seasons, the five phases, seasonal factors, internal organs, and their corresponding shen and virtues. The insight of these resonances begins with the following explanation:

> Nature contains the four seasons and the five phases of wood, fire, earth, metal, and water. The five phases interact, change, and transform

to create cold, summer heat, damp, dryness, and wind. The weather affects everything in the natural world and is the foundation for the cycle of life: birth, growth, maturation, and death. In the human body there are the five yin (zang) internal organs of the Heart, Spleen, Lungs, Kidneys, and the Liver. The organs provide the structure and the qi to form and allow the manifestation of the five spirits, which then gives rise to the five natural virtues and emotions.[14]

This is the unfolding of the five shen (five spirits) in the body. This explanation expresses the relationship between the cosmos and humanity: the macrocosm and microcosm. Chapter 8 of the *Ling Shu* presents the five shen and their relationships to the five Yin organs. Psychological, emotional, and mental functions of each organ are presented. The condition of the organs can influence the five shen, and their aspects of life. The condition of the five shen can also influence the organs. For example, fear can manifest if someone has chronic Kidney deficiency. If a person is under constant stress, the Liver can become stagnant and cause anger and irritability. This imbalanced condition can cause the Liver and its corresponding shen's (hun) imbalance to move into the divergent channel pathways. The divergent channels can assist in releasing the imbalances from the body.

Five shen resonances (correspondences) tell us much about the nature of the five shen. Here are the main resonances from the chapters "Roots and Spirit" and "The Manifestation of Yin and Yang from the Macrocosm to the Microcosm." These resonances are used in clinical practice. They are also the building blocks of the Five Shen Nei Dan practice.

RESONANCES
The twelve organs

- The Heart is the sovereign of all organs and represents the consciousness of one's spirit. It is responsible for intelligence, wisdom, and spiritual transformation.

- The Lung is the advisor. It helps the Heart in regulating the qi.

- The Liver is like the general. It is intelligent and courageous.

- The Gallbladder is like a judge. It has power of discrimination.
- The Pericardium is like the court jester. He makes the emperor laugh, bringing joy.
- The Stomach and Spleen are like warehouses; they store food and essences. They digest, transform, and transport food and nutrients.
- The Large Intestine transports turbidity (waste products).
- The Small Intestine receives the food that has been digested by the Spleen and Stomach; it further extracts, absorbs, and transports the food's essences from the extraction process throughout the body. It separates the pure from the turbid.
- The Kidneys store vitality. This mobilizes the four extremities. The Kidneys also benefit the memory, willpower, and coordination.
- The San Jiao promotes the transformation and transportation of fluids throughout the body.
- The Bladder is where water converges and is eliminated.

The five storehouses

- The Liver is the storehouse of blood, and the shelter of the human soul (hun spirit).
- The Spleen is the storehouse of nourishment, and the shelter of thought (yi spirit).
- The Heart is the storehouse for the channels, and the shelter of the spirit (shen spirit).
- The Lung is the storehouse of qi, and the shelter of the animal spirit (po spirit).
- The Kidneys are the storehouse of the seminal essence, and the shelter of the will (zhi spirit).

The five shen and their inherent qualities

- The spirit of the Heart is called the shen, and it rules mental and creative functions.
- The spirit of the Liver is called the hun, and it rules the nervous system and gives rise to extrasensory awareness.
- The spirit of the Spleen is known as the yi, and it rules logic or rational thought.
- The spirit of the Lungs is called the po, and it rules the animalistic instincts, and physical strength and endurance.
- The spirit of the Kidneys is called the zhi, and it rules the will, drive, ambition, and the survival instinct.

The five shen and emotions

- Anger can injure the Liver; but sadness can relieve anger. *Metal controls wood. The po controls the hun.*
- Too much joy can cause a depletion of the Heart qi. This can be counterbalanced by fear. *Water controls fire. The zhi controls the shen.*
- Excessive worry will deplete Spleen qi; but anger can restrain this worry. *Wood controls earth. The hun controls the yi.*
- Extreme grief can injure the Lungs; but it may be countered by the emotion of happiness. *Fire controls metal. The shen controls the po.*
- Fear and fright will damage the Kidneys. It can be defeated with understanding, logic, and rational thinking. *Earth controls water. The yi controls the zhi.*

In these five-phase relationships, the controlling cycle is identified to treat an imbalance. In my experience, when the controlling cycle is in balance, the controlling phase *shapes* the controlled phase. For example, the zhi (water) shapes the shen (fire). It shapes by sending its balanced energy and its virtues to the Heart shen, bringing it into balance. This shaping occurs for all the five shen. This process is a major aspect of the nei dan meditation presented in this book.

Some practitioners apply this controlling (shaping) theory to the five transporting points to treat emotional conditions. The Han dynasty classic medical text, the *Nan Ching—The Classic of Difficulties*, introduces the five phases points (the five element points); they are not presented in the *Su Wen* or the *Ling Shu*. In this method, the imbalanced organ is identified, and its controlling phase is needled. For example, if a person has anger and is irritable, the metal point on the Liver channel is treated. Liver 4, Middle Seal, is the metal point on the Liver channel. This point is treated to relieve anger. Anger can injure the Liver, but sadness can relieve anger. Sadness is the emotion of the Lungs, which is metal. Metal can relieve anger.

The knowledge of each of the five shen has important clinical value. When there is an imbalance of these emotions, match the emotion to its corresponding organ and shen. These connections are the foundation for an organ and five shen diagnosis. And it provides the basis for channel and acupuncture point selection.

The following insight from the *Ling Shu*, Chapter 8, "Roots and Spirit," is important in clinical practice:

> When the Heart and mind is frightened and full of distressed thoughts and anxiety, it can result in injury to the spirit. This can result in fear and *loss of self*.[15]

This quote expresses the view that, with stress and emotional turmoil, we can lose our connection of self, which is our spirit. Acupuncture can assist in clearing or releasing the emotional attachment to the turmoil. The release can assist in reconnecting to one's spirit; this process is sometimes called self-realization. The Five Shen Nei Dan meditation in this book assists in this process.

THE FIVE SHEN

The five shen are an example of the ancient Chinese awareness of the unity of the body, mind, and spirit. Five shen correspondences of the internal organs are presented in the *Su Wen*, Chapter 5, "The Manifestation of Yin and Yang from the Macrocosm to the Microcosm," and Chapter 8, "The

Sacred Teachings." This information is essential in making a diagnosis and developing a treatment plan. The key is to identify imbalances and the conditions that cause them. Often the emotional, psychological, and spiritual condition reveals areas of life that a person needs to understand in order to grow. It is common for a person to act in a way that causes the imbalances to be expressed in their life; this expression may be necessary to bring awareness of the condition. The awareness provides an opportunity to bring consciousness of the situation and begin a path of change and transformation. The practice of Chinese medicine, including acupuncture, herbs, and Qi Gong, can assist in this path of change, transformation, and self-realization.

The shen

The Heart houses the shen, which is the original spirit. Methods that connect a person to their Heart shen can provide the opportunity to realize knowledge, inspiration, wisdom, and guidance regarding the unity of life. Attuning to the Heart shen can allow direct experience of spirit, and the inseparable nature of the universe; this unity exists for all people. In Chinese culture, living from this awareness is called Wu Wei, which can be translated as "nothing extra." It is sometimes translated as "no-thing." Nothing extra means we add no extra stress, anxiety, opinions, beliefs, and preconceived ideas to our life. To live in the Tao is to live from our spirit, and the way to do this is by living in Wu Wei.

From an acupuncture pathway viewpoint, the chong and Kidney channels connect the Kidneys and the Heart, which is jing–shen, and Shao Yin. This channel flow reveals that there is a circuit of channels that are a pathway to the Heart shen, and the Heart shen can be accessed at any time. As healthcare practitioners, we can assist in helping our patients realize their shen (self-realization) by treating this channel circuit.

The shen includes the Small Intestine and Heart's innate quality of pursuing our quest in life. It can include things that allow a person to become more outgoing and more involved in overt expression. This expression allows one to access, attune, and express their yuan shen. And in this expression there is often a realization of the unity of life, which can be a transcendental experience. With time this unity of life becomes normal and a part of everyday life. Stagnation, blockages, and repressions of this aspect of our life can manifest in intense outward expressions, which can be physical or emotional. For example, yelling, screaming, punching, or emotional outbursts can occur at any time, reflecting the volatile and explosive nature of fire.

The Heart opens to the tongue. Shen imbalances can manifest in speech, which can include the inability to express oneself; the imbalance can include talking too much. Stagnations and repressions of the Heart shen can manifest in the chest, eyes, arms, and shoulders, causing a loss of the desire for outward movement and interaction in life. This can lead to a loss of the passion for life. It can also lead to bitterness (the taste and quality of the Heart). Connecting to our Heart shen is a primary experience in spiritual traditions. As practitioners of the healing arts, assisting others in making this connection or realization is one of the most powerful and life-changing experiences for both the practitioner and the patient.

The zhi

The Kidneys house the zhi shen, which corresponds to jing, and genetics (including ancestral influences). Ancestral medicine is the oldest historically based medicine in China. It originates in the Shang dynasty, at which time the Chinese viewed the living and the deceased as existing simultaneously, and therefore they influenced each other. A modern view of this influence can be genetics. It can also include the culture, religion, and beliefs of family, caretakers, and those with an influence on early life. Transcending any unfavorable influences is essential to living a fulfilling life. If they are not transcended they can lead to increased stagnation and rigidity.

Zhi relates to willpower. It includes the will and power to follow one's destiny. The Kidneys loathe cold, which can freeze water and change its essential nature and its ability to adapt to all situations. The Kidneys channel flows up the anterior of the body to the chest, creating the front shu points. These points are called the twelve shu points of the chest (Chapter 58 of the *Su Wen*). This pathway is one example of zhi seeking shen. It is the built-in energetic system in each person. If there is a freezing or rigidity due to ancestral influences, we may not be able to fulfill our destiny. The freezing (the ancestral and early life influences) can change the flowing and adaptive nature of each person. A goal in life should be to allow expression of the issues related to the freezing of our zhi. Allowing expression is letting go: by letting go we allow a space to appear, and this space is the place of change and transformation. Chapter 11 of the *Tao Te Ching* expresses this subtle truth:

> Thirty spokes together make a wheel for a cart.
> It is the empty space in the center of the wheel which enables it to be used.
> Mold clay in a vessel;
> It is the emptiness within that creates the usefulness of the vessel.
> Cut out doors and windows in a house;
> It is the empty space inside that creates the usefulness of the house.
> Thus, what we have may be something substantial,
> But its usefulness lies in the unoccupied, empty space.
> The substance of your body is enlivened by maintaining the part of you that is unoccupied.[16]

The zhi and jing represent unlimited possibilities. In Chinese philosophy, we call this "chaos" or Wu Ji, which is a state or energy field where anything is possible, and anything can manifest. It is a field of spontaneity. No limits are placed on it. This space is inside each person. When we live from this space, there is no freezing or rigidity placed on the Kidneys, jing, and zhi (the organ, substance, and shen). If our ancestral influence (genes) or our family post-natal influences freeze or block our ability to be open to all possibilities, our Kidneys and zhi will be unfavorably affected. This situation will require unblocking these blockages. Treatment and cultivation to allow expression of this aspect of life, which can be viewed as burning karma (Taoists may call it cause and effect), can allow one to become aware of the essential or primary nature of zhi. This awareness can facilitate unblocking other stagnations of the five shen, allowing self-realization. For the healthcare practitioner, this process can be supported with natural healing.

The Kidneys, water, and zhi contain a blueprint of life, or a destiny code. Allowing the zhi to unfold is fulfilling one's destiny. Internal alchemy can be viewed as accelerating personal development. When one is involved in activities (for instance, a profession, hobbies, exercise, dance, Qi Gong, Nei Gong, yoga, writing, or singing), they can allow immersion into these energetics and expression. This creates the possibility of accelerating the unfolding process (by expression).

The Kidneys open to the ears. Zhi imbalances can manifest in hearing conditions—not only diminished hearing, but also not hearing or understanding what others are saying.

The hun

The Liver houses the hun, which corresponds to the ethereal shen. The hun relates to the collective consciousness, and is the "we" aspect of consciousness or awareness. A person with wood/hun imbalances could mean that they need to allow expression in working with others for the benefit of the community, society, or the collective. This expression can include putting oneself in situations that allow concerns for others to manifest, which allows an awareness of this situation, and the opportunity to learn about it and grow. If a person has been in an environment that blocks that expression, they may act in a way that is contrary to their temperament. This can be acting in a selfish way, which is the opposite of unity and community. A treatment plan for this person can be to unblock the areas of stagnation to allow expression related to the hun temperament. The divergent channels can assist in releasing this Liver hun suppression.

Balance is key in Chinese medicine. Our shen temperament needs to be balanced. If one's expression is extreme, it is not balanced, and can lead to pathological patterns. If hun qualities are expressed to an extreme, one can be too attached to the collective and other people, at the cost of taking care of oneself and one's own health and well-being. In a way, such people are rejecting their life and taking on the extreme wood nature of rising and flying away, which can be an escape from their body or their life. A balanced expression is key in providing the environment for a healthy unfolding of one's life path.

The Liver and hun relate to planning and thinking of the future, and how to achieve goals. If there is an extreme or imbalanced quality within these aspects of a person, we can consider it a hun condition. We can then develop a treatment plan to clear the blockages in the body and channels that may contribute to the imbalance. When the blockage is removed, focus can be on treatment and cultivation that allows a natural expression of the constitutional temperament.

The Liver opens to the eyes. Hun imbalances can manifest in seeing problems, diminished eyesight, or lack of perceiving. This can be lack of insight, or inner seeing, and not just physical vision.

The po

The Lungs house the po, which corresponds to the corporeal shen. The po relates to the physical body. The correspondences include the senses, desires, and the emotions. Imbalances in the po can manifest as over-attachments in those areas of life. The po can be expressed in selfishness. It's the "me, me, me" aspect of self. When the po is imbalanced, focus is directed on the desire for physical and self-pleasure. Selfishness and greediness can be part of a po disharmony.

The Large Intestine is the only primary channel that crosses the midline of the body. Some refer to it as the channel of polarity. A polarized po is a common condition in modern society. Loneliness is a common condition of the imbalanced po. Part of this comes from its ability to polarize itself, causing a separation from others, society, the creator, and life itself. Out of this polarity comes isolation, separation, and intensified loneliness. These imbalanced experiences and emotions can cause a response to the polarization that can initiate change. Loneliness and unhappiness can lead a person to seek another way to live and experience life; the driving force is the body's innate intelligence to seek homeostasis. The practitioner can develop a treatment plan to release the intensities of an imbalanced po. The treatment can include a connecting channel (luo channel) treatment to release the emotions, and a divergent channel treatment on the Lungs and Large Intestine channels can assist in the release.

A balanced po seeks a healthy expression of enjoying the physical body. When the po is imbalanced it can be expressed in being selfish, greedy, and neglecting or ignoring one's body. The Lungs are connected to the nose. Breathing is a key to bringing the po into the present moment, freeing one from the polarity of the po. There is no polarity or separation in the current moment: polarity only occurs in the thoughts of the past or future. Polarity creates separation, isolation, and loneliness. Breathing practices, including Qi Gong and Tai Chi Chuan, are traditional ways that can regulate the breath, calm the po, and promote balance.

The yi

The Spleen houses the yi shen. The yi corresponds to the intellect, thoughts, concepts, and ideas. The element of the Spleen is earth. Grounding, organizing, and digestion are qualities of the earth, Spleen, and the Stomach. The Spleen corresponds to the mouth, which processes food and drink, and transforms them into nutritive substances. The condition of the Spleen and the Stomach directly influences that transformation process. Transforming food and drink is the physical transformation. The earth organs, the Spleen and Stomach, also are involved in the psycho-emotional transformation process. Similar to how food and drink goes into the mouth (Spleen and Stomach) to be processed and transformed, all experiences in life are processed by the yi. The yi processes our life experiences; it organizes, categorizes, filters, and makes sense of our experiences. In the same way that the condition of the Spleen and the Stomach determines the quality of the nutrition processed from digesting food, the condition of the yi is instrumental in the processing of our experiences in life, and our emotional well-being.

The condition of our yi, which includes the way we perceive, experience, and process life, influences the hun, po, zhi, and shen. The yi includes our thinking and opinions about people and life. If the yi is in an imbalanced or unhealthy state, all the five shen and their correspondences are influenced. The yi, as the transformer, processes our experiences. The yi includes the intellect and thoughts. When these qualities are over-developed, the other aspects of our body, mind, and spirit become imbalanced. When the yi is imbalanced, we become rigid and narrow, and respond to life in a conditioned way. We respond to life based on our past experiences. However, often the past understanding is rooted in fear, anger, misunderstandings, and prejudice; these influences create a conditioned response. The yi is susceptible to fixed, rigid, and repetitive patterns and reactions based on past experiences. One reason is that the Spleen, and therefore the yi, has a function of holding. The Spleen holds blood in the vessels. The yi holds as well. It holds emotions and thoughts in the blood. This holding function explains how the yi holds on to experiences, and how we can live in these held experiences, living in the past.

The yi includes mindfulness. What we place attention on and retain in our mind is mindfulness. The yi can be overwhelmed by experiences, especially when we are at a young age and not capable of dealing with them. The yi can go into survival mode and create patterns of behavior to survive that can become our constitution, our reactive ways of responding to life. These imprints need to be understood so we can be released from their influence and allow an openness to the spontaneity of life. Becoming open to life as it is, not what it should be, not what it must be, or not as we desire it to be, allows us to live from our shen. Living from our shen allows us to live in the present moment, and in a spontaneous way.

The yi can be imbalanced when one is too attached to thoughts and emotions; a person can become trapped in them. They are generally caught in past experiences, or they are worrying about the future. They tend to suffer from repetitive and obsessive thoughts and thinking due to the inability to let go. Not being able to let go prevents one from living in the present moment. Feelings can be viewed as normal, natural aspects of life—they are spontaneous; but an imbalanced yi can try to hold on to these feelings. This process is trying to artificially retain something that should be experienced and allowed to leave, like the way the sun and the moon flow in endless cycles of waxing and waning. This *trying* creates a separation from fully experiencing the present moment. The imbalanced yi will hold and maintain past experiences, keeping them alive by continual thinking. Viewing these feelings as wei or superficial energetics is Yang. This energetic quality includes the natural flow of appearing and leaving. To keep these feelings alive takes Yin, which has the quality to store and maintain. The Spleen and the yi's Yin quality is blood. By continual thinking about feelings or experiences, the Spleen's energetics transforms them into emotions, which are then stored in the blood. This process illustrates how we keep emotions alive. What we hold is not the real experience; it is a thought or memory. This holding process becomes part of conditioning, and eventually our constitution, and the inability to live in a spontaneous way.

The yi corresponds to earth, which has the qualities of being rooted and grounded. The yi also includes the Stomach and Spleen's innate qualities of being grounded in one's choices and actions, creating attitudes of life based on being comfortable with them. Stagnations in these areas prevent a person from allowing new viewpoints, understandings, choices, and actions. These stagnations prevent us from letting go of the past, preventing the ability to experience life in a spontaneous way. Dampness and phlegm can manifest from these stagnations, creating blockages and a rigidity against seeing new things in life. Damp and phlegm can be viewed as the physical manifestation of concepts and thoughts that slow us down and stagnate us.

The Spleen opens to the mouth. Yi imbalances can manifest in eating disorders because imbalances of the Spleen/Stomach and the yi/mouth can be expressed in the mouth and eating.

The imbalances of the five shen, especially the emotions, can transfer to any of the acupuncture channels. For example, anger can influence the muscle channels, which influences posture and the musculo-skeletal system. Anger can be held in the connecting channels, intensifying emotions. Anger can also influence the primary channels and the functions of the organs. It is common for anger to influence digestion. This is wood overacting on earth. Anger can transfer into the divergent channels, causing stagnations and pain in these channels. And when anger becomes an ongoing and chronic experience, it can enter the eight extraordinary channels and become part of the constitution. The process of the emotion anger transferring to other channel systems reflects the interdependence of the channel system.

FIVE SHEN GROUP DYNAMICS

The five shen is a model that can become the basis of diagnosis and treatment plans. When the five shen correspondences become familiar, their imbalances become clear. The root of an imbalance can originate from a variety of sources, including pre-natal and post-natal influences.

It is important to view the five shen as five aspects of one shen (a person). Each of the five shen contains unique aspects of a person. And each shen shapes other shen in a way required for a person to be whole. The five phases cycles illustrate important relationships within the five shen. Figure 7.1 depicts the five shen in circular formation. When the controlling (ko) cycle is in balance, it is a harmonizing force. When there is an imbalance it can create unfavorable conditions; it can be overacting. The organs/shen contain an innate intelligence, which contains a message to be sent to its related shen (it provides an integral aspect of the functioning of its partner). The five phases cycles are the patterns for these integral relationships.

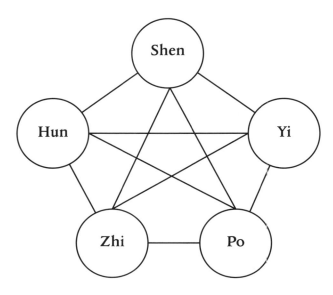

Figure 7.1 The five shen

The five shen (five phases) cycles contain a shaping or message-sharing function. For example, the Heart shen or fire has a controlling or shaping relationship with the Lungs and the po. The Heart shen sends its energy or message to the po. The message from the Heart shen to the Lung po is that we are essentially spirit. This realization guides the po spirit in its expression of the physical aspect of life. The po qualities are close to the physical body, the physical aspect of life. When it is imbalanced it is susceptible to being polarized, creating imbalances that can manifest as selfishness. This selfishness can include an unhealthy pursuit of one's own needs, desires, and pleasures, often ignoring other people's needs. It's the Heart shen that expresses to the po its original nature, the yuan shen. The balance of the two allows for the smooth expression of po in life. This expression is guided by the Heart shen. When the shen and the po are in balance, this interaction and exchange is always occurring. When we create a life that maintains this relationship, our experience is a natural, spontaneous expression of spirit. It can be called living in the Tao, or living in spirit. Spiritual traditions around the world call it Christ consciousness, Krishna consciousness, or Buddha nature.

The po and hun

The po shen contains the innate intelligence of the importance of living in this world, enjoying it, and allowing full expression of our life in the here and now. The po sends this message to the hun spirit (metal controlling or shaping wood), which is the ethereal spirit. The hun includes the collective aspect of our life. This is the aspect of our life that we experience when we are attuned to the whole, part of a collective society and a unified universe.

When the hun is imbalanced it can include a denial of the physical body; this can be when a person pursues a spiritual direction in an attempt to deny the physical body and life. If there is a rejection of the physical body and life, a deep polarization can occur. The imbalanced hun can be too involved in society or assisting others to the detriment of their own health. One may believe it is of greater value to help others, but if it is a denial of a healthy enjoyment of their physical life and body then it is a rejection of their physical needs and desires. This rejection can create a polarity and separation, which creates an imbalance not only of the po and hun, but also of the other shen. The po–hun relationship includes the balanced relationship between self and others, and the individual and society.

The hun and yi

The hun contains the innate intelligence of the collective aspect of life. The hun sends this message to the yi, the Spleen's shen. This interaction is wood shaping or influencing earth. The yi contains our conceptual or intellectual capabilities. This is our ability to reason, be logical, and organize and categorize; it includes intention (focus). The Spleen and the yi process not only food and drink but also our experiences of life. When the yi is imbalanced it can lead to separation of oneself from other people and society, creating isolation and polarization.

Being too attached to thoughts and concepts turns a person's attention from real life, which creates a schism, because the body innately knows there is one reality. The reality is living in the present. Additionally, an imbalanced yi can manifest as obsessive and repetitive actions. These actions may be rooted in an extreme or distorted understanding or perception of experiences or thoughts. The hun can send its energy and message to the yi: the message is that we are part of the whole, not separate from the whole of life. Yi qualities are just one aspect of a person and not the primary aspect. The hun can help balance the yi to receive and process life in a clear, spontaneous way, and not in a conditioned, repetitive way.

The yi and zhi

The yi or earth shapes or sends a message to the zhi, the shen of the Kidneys. The zhi contains an innate intelligence of our unlimited nature, the capacity to become anything: this is called "chaos" in Taoist philosophy; it is our primordial nature. It is before thinking, before the dualistic categorization of all things in life. When this aspect of our life is over-developed, we become conditioned in how we respond to people, activities, and situations. An imbalanced yi can have a significant influence on the zhi. It can overact on it, forcing it into a specific shape, which can prevent its natural free-flowing nature from being expressed.

The zhi contains willpower, the will and power to achieve goals and objectives. It is also the will and power to live the type of life we desire. One variation of this is the will and desire to seek our true nature, and then live from it. Zhi corresponds to water. Water's nature includes taking any form or shape; it is the flexibility to adapt to all situations. The zhi loathes cold. One reason for this is that cold freezes water, changing its innate nature of adaptability. The yi can help shape the zhi to accomplish goals and objectives. One way it does this is by applying *focus* on achieving or accomplishing.

The zhi needs some direction or focus, or it can spread itself too much and not accomplish. The relationship between the yi and the zhi, earth and water, and the pre-natal and post-natal, can be found in many aspects of Chinese medicine. One interesting relationship is between the chong channel and the Spleen and Stomach. The chong channel begins at chong qi, Stomach 30. The Stomach channel is earth, and this pathway connection illustrates earth shaping the form of jing as it unfolds in life. Additionally, gongsun, Spleen 4, is the opening point of the chong channel; this relationship is also earth shaping water. It is the post-natal shaping pre-natal.

A balanced yi provides a favorable focus and intention that allows the zhi to unfold in a healthy way. If the yi is imbalanced it can cause rigid thinking and actions, and can create repetitive and obsessive activities. The zhi needs the yi to have an openness to receive and experience life. Openness allows the zhi to maintain the ability to be flexible and adaptive. The zhi needs this to allow its natural unfolding and the fulfillment of one's destiny.

The zhi and shen

The zhi or water shapes and sends its energy to the Heart shen. This relationship is the classic Chinese model of Yin–Yang, water–fire, Shao Yin, and jing–shen. This relationship can be viewed as the zhi's capacity to become anything. There is a clear direction within all these possibilities: it is jing seeking shen, the zhi seeking the Heart shen. The Kidney's external pathway, the pathway where the points are located, flows past the Heart area and contains the front shu points. These five points have a profound influence on the five shen. The points are presented in Chapter 58 of the *Su Wen*, "The Acupuncture Points."

The Heart shen contains our true nature. Some traditions view realization of this aspect of our nature as the primary goal or purpose of life. This realization provides the opportunity to live from this awareness. Jing seeking shen can be viewed as our quest in life. The models of jing–shen, water–fire, and Yin–Yang, along with the trajectory connections between the Kidneys and Heart, show the inner energetic system reflecting this quest.

The divergent channels can assist in clearing away the rough preventing spiritual realization. They can also guide one's awareness of their spirit. In this way, a divergent channel treatment offers a way to support spiritual realization.

Table 7.1 summarizes fundamental information about the five shen. This information can be used to make a five shen diagnosis.

Table 7.1 Five shen and correspondences

Zhi Water	Kidneys Bladder	Lineage, genetics, willpower, reproduction, vision, dreams, destiny, unlimited possibilities, destiny code, the will to live your destiny
Hun Wood	Liver Gallbladder	Collective, intelligence, growth, cultivation, direction, ethereal, planning, decision making, judgments
Shen Fire	Heart Small Intestine	Spirit, consciousness, quest, guidance, intuition, wisdom, yuan shen, true spirit
Yi Earth	Spleen Stomach	Concepts, thoughts, intellect, grounding, rooting, practical, digesting life experiences, organizing, holding emotions/thoughts/blood, mindfulness, polarity, separation
Po Metal	Lungs Large Intestine	Physical body, physical desires, sensitivity to emotions, selfishness, isolation, inability to forgive

CHAPTER 8

THE NINE NEEDLES

THE NINE NEEDLES AND THE PRACTICE OF ACUPUNCTURE

Acupuncture based on the *Ling Shu* is a sophisticated and complete system of healing. In the modern practice of acupuncture it is common to use only a few methods and applications from this Han dynasty classic. By following the guidance of the ancient practitioners we can incorporate their insights and clinical experience into the modern practice of acupuncture. "The Nine Needles" contains more than insight and application; it contains a theoretical foundation for understanding the acupuncture channel system.

Mirroring the body, the acupuncture channel system contains layers. Each channel layer corresponds to vital substances, pathogens, and pathology. The *Su Wen* and the *Ling Shu* describe the vital substances, pathology, and needling methods to treat the different channel systems. This can assist the modern practitioner in applying more effective methods in clinical practice.

There are many references in the *Su Wen* and the *Ling Shu* regarding the locations or depths of the different channels. The following references describe the acupuncture layering system, reflecting that there is a channel system that is distributed throughout the body. Treating the proper channel system can more effectively treat conditions than using one channel system to treat all conditions. For example, it is common for modern practitioners to use the primary channels to treat most conditions. The classics advise us to consider which of the five channel systems to use for a treatment, and not to use only the primary channels:

In general, when a pathogen invades the body, it first enters the skin level. If it lingers, or is not expelled, it will travel into the Micro Luo. If it is not expelled it will travel to the regular luo channels, if it is not expelled it moves to the main channels and then the internal organs. This is the progression of a pathogen from the skin level into the organs.[17]

It is said the illness may be on the hair level, the skin level, the muscle level, the level of channels, the tendon level, and bone and marrow level. When treating the hair level do not damage the skin level. If the illness is at the skin level do not damage the muscle level, if the illness is at the muscle level needling too deeply will damage the channel level. In illness of the tendons needling too deeply will damage the bone level, in illness of the bones needling too deeply will damage the marrow.[18]

These *Su Wen* references provide the framework for the correlation between pathogens, pathology, channels, needles, and needling techniques for applications of the nine needles. The channel system can be viewed with the cutaneous regions at the superficial or wei layer, and the eight extraordinary channels at the deep or yuan layer:

Superficial or Wei Layer

Cutaneous regions (wei layer)
Tendon muscle (wei layer)
Luo channels (wei layer)
Primary channels (ying layer)
Divergent channels (wei, ying, yuan layers)
Eight extraordinary channels (yuan layer)

Deep or Yuan Layer

The early Chinese medical practitioners developed needles and techniques that corresponded with each channel system, and their pathology. When the channel system and its pathology are treated with the nine needles, or a treatment/stimulation method that reflects the effects of a needling method, a comprehensive method for the practice of acupuncture is being applied in clinical practice. Throughout the long history of the practice of acupuncture, practitioners reduced the number of needles. In an attempt to mimic the effects of the different needles, practitioners developed numerous needling methods and techniques. These methods offer a way to obtain specific effects with fewer needles.

Chapter 1 of the *Ling Shu*, "Of Nine Needles and the Twelve Source Points," presents a framework for how the acupuncture system is one unified system. Each of the needles influences a certain channel and anatomical area. The needling methods cause a certain reaction in the channel system. Because the channel system is integrated, channels can influence other channels. A unique aspect of the divergent channels is that they connect to and can influence all the channel systems. They can be used to support any of the channels, and they can support a treatment plan, including the clinical objective of the needles and the methods applied in a treatment. For example, if the treatment plan is to reinforce the Spleen and the Stomach, the divergent channels can be reinforced to increase the body's ability to guide qi to the Spleen and the Stomach. It does this by stimulating more channels and vital substances then treating only the Spleen and Stomach primary channels. The divergent channels stimulate, gather, and guide the body's channels and vital substances to support the targeted channels, organs, and areas of the body. This additional influence assists in restoring the channel or organ system. This treatment method allows for a more effective way to utilize the body's channel system and vital substances and is a potent part of the clinical applications of the divergent channels.

THE NINE NEEDLES

The nine needles are presented in the *Su Wen,* Chapter 54, "The Art of Acupuncture," and Chapter 50, "Rudiments of Acupuncture"; and in the *Ling Shu,* Chapter 1, "Of Nine Needles and the Twelve Source Points," and Chapter 7, "On Governing the Needles." The names, descriptions, sizes, needling methods, and the pathogens the nine needles treat is now presented.

THE DIVERGENT CHANNELS—JING BIE

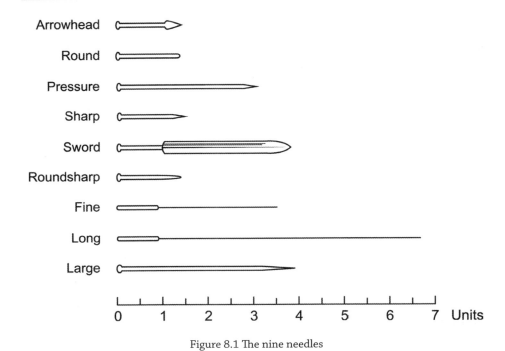

Figure 8.1 The nine needles

1. Arrowhead/Chisel/Seven star, Chanzhen, 1.6 cun

This needle is used on the superficial layers. It arouses Yang Qi and stimulates wei qi to release exterior pathogenic factors.

The technique is like chiseling forward, moving one way continually deeper as the needle is pushed along the body.

The needle is used for the muscle (sinew) channels. It is effective when cold causes a binding of the channels. It can treat cold in the joints. It is effective in releasing pathogens influencing the Lungs.

2. Round, Yuanzhen, 1.6 cun

This needle influences stasis of the sinews. The technique creates circular movements to hook the needle to separate the muscles. Applying this method includes positioning the patient to allow muscles to separate. The needle looks like a spoon, which can move in between the muscles to separate them, creating a space to scoop out the pathogens.

This needle is good for treating wind in the sinew channels. It can relax the muscles. Performing gua sha after using the round needle can promote bringing wind and pathogens to the surface to be released.

3. Pressure/Spoon, Tizhen, 3.5 cun

The spoon needle is like a round needle; it is dull at the end and is used for scraping and rubbing, similar to gua sha. The practitioner can scrape the head of the needle. This needle arouses qi.

The technique for this needle is the shaking needle method. Emphasis is on the wrist. The massage or tui na method is friction, which pushes qi to the extremities.

4. Sharp/Lance/Three edged, Fengzhen, 1.6 cun

This needle is for treating the connecting/luo/blood channels. It is used to bleed. It especially treats chronic bi syndrome. It can drain blood from the five zang organs and it can release toxins. It can treat chronic conditions and blood stasis. Applications include treating luo points.

This is contraindicated in the winter. The winter is for storage and not releasing. It is advised to use fewer points in the winter as the body is trying to hibernate and store to rejuvenate.

5. Sword, Pizhen, 4 cun

This needle influences the ying or blood level. It can drain pustule eruptions, abscesses, boils, swellings, and febrile conditions.

The method is cutting. This method includes stimulating by moving backward and forward.

6. Roundsharp/Sharp, Yuanlizhen, 1.6 cun

This is the common filiform needle used today. This needle can grasp the qi (it can capture the qi of the body).

It is used for the primary channels, and conditions of the internal organs. It can also treat acute, sudden bi obstruction.

7. Fine, Haozhen, 3.6 cun

This needle is long and can be used for shallow needling and threading points together.

One method is to pinch the skin to provide space, pinch as you slide along the skin as you thread, and pinch and hold as you slide from one point to another.

The needle is for cutaneous and dermatological conditions.

8. Long, Changzhen, 7 cun

This needle treats deep-level conditions. The long needle influences Yang Qi, cold, and wind cold in the Tai Yin channels. It is used for paralysis, numbness, and pain. This needle can access deep areas where cold is trapped, which includes the joints and bones. It allows accessing the center or deep regions, and it can warm the center of the body, including the abdomen.

9. Large/Big, Dazhen, 4 cun

This needle can treat the eight extraordinary and the divergent channels. It is long enough to enter the deep/yuan layers.

It can be used to treat joints, swellings, edema, damp, and wind-damp-cold. It can open gates of the body, for example the small articulations.

Table 8.1 lists the nine needles, with their name, size, and a brief description of each needle.

Table 8.1 Nine needles summary

Number	Needle	Name	Size
1	Arrowhead Chisel Seven star	Chanzhen	A big head with a sharp tip 1.6 cun
2	Round	Yuanzhen	A round body and a head like an egg 1.6 cun
3	Pressure Spoon	Tizhen	A sharp tip like a grain of millet 3.5 cun
4	Sharp Lance Three edged	Fengzhen	Three cutting edges 1.6 cun
5	Sword	Pizhen	A sharp tip like a sword 4 cun
6	Roundsharp Sharp	Yuanlizhen	A sharp tip like hair and its body a bit larger 1.6 cun
7	Fine	Haozhen	A tip like a mosquito's beak 3.6 cun
8	Long	Changzhen	A sharp tip and thin body 7 cun
9	Large Big	Dazhen	A tip like a stick and slightly round 4 cun

Table 8.2 presents the channel system with the corresponding vital substance, area of influence, and the needles that treat them.

Table 8.2 The nine needles and the channels of acupuncture

Channel	Substances	Major area of influence	Needle
Sinew	Wei qi	Superficial anatomy	Arrowhead/Chisel/Seven star Round Pressure/Spoon
Luo	Ying/Blood	Emotions	Pressure/Spoon Lance/Sharp, Roundsharp
Primary	Wei qi Ying qi	Internal organs	Roundsharp/Sharp Sword
Divergent	Wei qi Yuan qi	Surface-deep	Long Large/Big
Eight extraordinary	Jing Yuan qi	Deepest levels Jing level	Long Large/Big

The nine needles and the basic areas they treat are presented in Table 8.3.

Table 8.3 The nine needles and the channels and conditions

Needle	Function
Arrowhead	Sinew channels, cutaneous conditions, releases pathogens from the Lungs
Round	Wind in the sinew channels
Pressure	Arouses qi
Sharp	Luo channels
Sword	Treats blood level, abscesses, boils, swellings, febrile conditions
Roundsharp	Primary channels, organs, acute bi syndrome
Fine	Cutaneous regions, dermatological conditions
Long	Divergent channels, deep areas of the body: joints/bones, abdomen
Large	Eight extraordinary and the divergent channels, joints, swellings

The nine needles provide a framework for viewing pathology in each of the channel systems. They also offer needling methods that effectively treat the individual channels and pathology in them. This is important because in modern clinical practice it is not common or practical to use all nine needles; however, we can apply a needling technique to mimic the action of the needle, which can cause an energetic reaction that mirrors each of the nine needles. Including a needling technique in treatments can enhance their effectiveness. This is one of the most significant insights of the early practitioners of acupuncture.

CHAPTER 9

GUIDING THEORIES AND PRINCIPLES

A goal of this book is to present classical Chinese medical theories and principles that assist in determining when the divergent channels would be effective in a treatment. The *Su Wen* and the *Ling Shu* present treatment strategies and methods for the clinical applications of acupuncture. There are three main acupuncture treatment strategies: reinforcing, reducing, and dredging (clearing stasis). There are also a variety of strategies for selecting channels and points. When strategies for selecting channels and points are combined with needling methods, the effectiveness of a treatment increases.

This chapter presents 14 Chinese medical theories, principles, and methods that can guide the practitioner to determine if the divergent channels would be an effective addition to a treatment plan. The twelve foundation principles are:

1. Three layers of the body
2. From beginning to end
3. The major channels
4. Yin–Yang paired channels and the transporting points
5. Entering and exiting
6. Roots and Ends
7. Fifty cycles
8. Anatomical structures and the divergent channels

9. Distal needling

10. Emotions and the divergent channels

11. Rivers and channels

12. The muscle channels

13. Measurements in reference to the bones

14. Needling technique methods

THREE LAYERS OF THE BODY

The *Ling Shu*, Chapter 1, "Of Nine Needles and the Twelve Source Points," and Chapter 2, "An Explanation of the Minute Needles," presents a variety of important aspects for the practice of acupuncture. One key insight revealed in these chapters is that the body can be viewed in three layers: the top, middle, and bottom (the wei, ying, and yuan layers). The vital substances or pathogens can be located in one or more of the three layers. Diagnosing where the condition is located is essential in an effective treatment. The wei layer includes the muscle (sinew) and connecting channels. The ying layer includes the primary channels. The yuan layer includes the eight extraordinary channels. The divergent channels connect to and influence the wei, ying, and yuan layers. The divergent channels' ability to influence all three layers is what makes this channel system unique. Targeting the specific layer where the condition is located, as well as its corresponding channel system(s), allows the practitioner to guide substances to an area (reinforce); guide pathogens away from an area (reduce); or clear stagnations (dredge). The divergent channels have the capacity to influence all three layers of the body, which makes them very useful in clinical practice.

Chapter 1 of the *Ling Shu* presents the nine needles. Each needle treats specific layers, pathogens, and channels. This is a sophisticated system of correspondences. The system is a guide to treating specific channels and specific pathogenic factors and conditions. For example, selecting the channel system(s) where the condition is located, selecting a corresponding needle, and inserting and stimulating the needle at the proper layer (channel system) are all part of a channel correspondence. This layering system shows how different conditions affect different channels, organs, and vital substances, and can most effectively be treated by using the appropriate technique. Learning to identify the layer/channel system where a condition is located is an essential aspect of an effective treatment plan.

FROM BEGINNING TO END

The *Ling Shu*, Chapter 9, "From Beginning to End," presents a variety of acupuncture theories and applications. There are two that relate to divergent channels theory and clinical applications. The first is the three depths of acupuncture. As described above, the depths or levels are the wei, ying, and yuan levels. It says the first depth is a shallow insertion (wei level), the second depth is a middle insertion (ying level), and the third depth is deep insertion (yuan level). This reference confirms Chapter 7, "On Governing the Needles," and its understanding of the three levels (presented later in this chapter). The three levels reveal how to influence the channel system. For example, to influence the superficial levels, which include the sinew, connecting, and divergent channels, needle shallowly. To influence the middle levels, which are the primary channels, needle to the middle level. And to treat the deep level, which includes the eight extraordinary and divergent channels, needle to the deep level. Needling the proper level is essential to obtain effective clinical results.

The *Ling Shu*, Chapter 9, also states that if the condition is located at the upper body, treat the lower body. And if the condition is at the lower body, treat the upper body. It also suggests, if the condition is at the head, treat the foot. And if the condition is at the loins, treat the crease of the knee. This reference is a guiding principle to contra-lateral needling. This type of needling is based on two principles: the first is the ability of one side of the body to treat the opposite side; and the second is an understanding that a condition can begin in one location and move to another location. If one is able to diagnose the origin of the condition, and it is perceived that the condition (pathogen) has moved to another location, needling contra-laterally is actually needling the origin of the condition. In clinical strategies, using the divergent channels, inserting the needles at the origin of the condition, and moving to the opposite side of the body provide an effective approach.

THE MAJOR CHANNELS

The *Ling Shu*, Chapter 10, "The Major Channels," presents the primary channels. This chapter includes their pathways. It does not list any acupuncture points (though some points are listed as point location references for the pathway). The chapter presents excess and deficiency conditions of the channels, and it includes the connecting channels. The chapter includes an understanding that conditions in each of the channels can be transferred to each other. Because the channel system is interwoven, pathogenic factors can move within the three levels of the body and their corresponding channels. The primary channels are in the middle position of the three levels. They can influence the deeper and superficial levels, which are below and above their level. Because the divergent channels arise from the primary channels, and connect to the superficial and deep levels, they are a bridge to influencing both levels in treatments.

YIN-YANG PAIRED CHANNELS AND THE TRANSPORTING POINTS

The *Ling Shu*, Chapter 2, "The Roots of the Acupuncture Points," presents the transporting points. These are the well, spring, stream, river, and sea points on each channel. The transporting points are one of the most powerful acupuncture point categories in the *Su Wen* and the *Ling Shu*. These points can treat any condition of the channel and organ and can be included as supplemental points to support a divergent channel treatment. In the *Ling Shu*, there are no five-phase points. This category of points was added in the *Nan Ching—The Classic of Difficulties*. From a *Ling Shu* perspective, there was no five-phase treatment using five-phase points (e.g., Lung 9 is a source and stream point—it is not an earth point); at that time a five-phase treatment would be treating five-phase channels. For example, if the Lungs were deficient, points on the Spleen or Stomach channel would be selected to reinforce the Lungs. This is earth reinforcing metal.

Chapter 2, "The Roots of the Acupuncture Points," also presents the Yin–Yang coupled paired primary channels and organs. The *Ling Shu* practitioners confirmed that these channels are connected and can influence each other. Pathogens can transfer from one channel to the other. Because they are pairs, they can be viewed as one interconnected channel, and they can treat each other. The *Ling Shu*, Chapter 9, "From Beginning to End," presents a method for how to use the Yin–Yang paired channels in treatments. Each treatment includes using Yin–Yang primary channel pairs. For example, if there is Stomach excess, points on the Stomach and Spleen channels would be included in the treatment. We can apply that same strategy to the divergent channels. Each divergent channel treatment can include using the Yin–Yang paired channels. A synergy is created when combining the divergent channel pairs.

ENTERING AND EXITING

The *Ling Shu*, Chapter 3, "An Explanation of the Minute Needles," presents a few important insights that relate to the clinical applications of the divergent channels. The first insight is knowing where qi enters and exits, and knowing the channels that are diseased:

> The spirit is the primary qi, the guest is the evil qi. Located at the door means the evil qi pursues the primary qi at those locations where the evil and the primary qi comes out and enters. Don't just stare at the disease. Begin by knowing the evil and the primary qi and which channels are diseased. For illness, know the origins. First know which channels are diseased, then treat them at those locations.[19]

Entering and exiting is another example of the *Ling Shu* practitioner's view of the importance of knowing the location of the condition (the channels system) in clinical practice.

ROOTS AND ENDS

The *Ling Shu*, Chapter 5, "Roots and Ends," presents two very important insights that contribute to clinical applications of the divergent channels. The following quote expresses these insights:

> There are an extraordinary number of diseases in the divergent (separate) channels. And they cannot be counted without knowing the roots and ends of the five organs and six bowels. Diseases can

break open the gates and upset the pivots and travel through the gates and inner doors. For one that comprehends ends and beginnings, one sentence is enough. For one that does not understand ends and beginnings, the way of the needle is completely cut off.[20]

The beginnings and ends are locations where the channels begin and end. Some of these locations are different than the standard beginnings based on the primary channels with the modern number system of the acupuncture points. The channels begin at their well point. They do not follow the common order of the channel flow based on the ying qi cycle (the daily meridian clock). The ends and beginnings are:

- Tai Yang has its root (beginning) at extreme Yin, Bladder 67, and ends at the eye (destiny door, Bladder 1).
- Yang Ming begins at tip exchange, Stomach 45, and ends at the great forehead (Stomach 8).
- Shao Yang begins at cavity of Yin, Gallbladder 44, and ends at the ear, at window basket (listening palace, Small Intestine 19).
- Tai Yin begins at hidden white, Spleen 1, and ends at the Stomach (ren zhong, Ren 12).
- Shao Yin begins at yong quan, Kidney 1, and ends at the throat (lingquan, Ren 23).
- Jue Yin begins at da dun, Liver 1, and ends at the chest (tan zhong, Ren 17).

The roots and ends are describing a path and range of the channels' flow. If we combine the original statement, that there are an extraordinary number of diseases in the divergent channels, along with the pathway descriptions, the writers are expressing that conditions of the channels can be transferred from and to the locations presented in the roots and endings. These locations can be treated when the areas along the roots and endings are affected. Table 9.1 summarizes the roots and ends.

Table 9.1 Roots and ends

Channel	Root begins	Ending ends	Anatomical area of the ending
Tai Yang	Bladder 67	Bladder 1	Eyes
Shao Yang	Gallbladder 44	Small Intestine 19	Ear
Yang Ming	Stomach 45	Stomach 8	Corner of the head
Tai Yin	Spleen 1	Ren 12	Stomach
Shao Yin	Kidney 1	Ren 23	Throat
Jue Yin	Liver 1	Ren 17	Chest

FIFTY CYCLES

The *Ling Shu*, Chapter 5, "Roots and Ends," also presents that nourishing (ying) qi circulates 50 times per day. If it does not circulate 50 times it reflects an imbalance of the channels and organs. The text states that this lack of normal circulation is the beginning of "chaos" (this chaos is different than the Wu Ji chaos explained earlier in Chapter 7), which reflects imbalances in the channels and organs, and leads to illness. The imbalances can follow the roots and endings flow, or the nourishing cycle (*Ling Shu*, Chapter 16, "The Nourishing Cycle") of the organs and channels. These channel patterns are maps that should be included in diagnosis and developing treatment plans. For example, if the Lungs are deficient and the ying qi cycle is affected, treat Ren 12, zhong wan. The nourishing qi cycle begins in the center of the Stomach (Ren 12, zhong wan), and eventually flows to the Lungs. When zhong wan is reinforced it reinforces the Lungs; it is earth reinforcing metal. They are also Tai Yin paired channels.

ANATOMICAL STRUCTURES AND THE DIVERGENT CHANNELS

The *Ling Shu*, Chapter 6, "Longevity or Premature Death, to be Hard or Soft," presents an important theory that plays an essential role in the clinical applications of the divergent channels. This chapter presents a relationship between anatomical structures of the body. The chapter states that internally there is Yin and Yang, and externally there is Yin and Yang. In the interior, the Yin (zang) organs are Yin, and the Yang (fu) organs are Yang. At the exterior, Yin is the bones, and Yang is the skin. When the bones and the skin are connected to their corresponding channels and vital substances, a set of relationships is revealed that can be applied to clinical applications of the divergent channels. The skin includes the exterior channels and their substances: the sinew channels and wei qi. The bones include the eight extraordinary channels, jing, and source qi.

These relationships indicate two clinical applications: the first is that channels that connect to the skin can influence the sinew channels and wei qi; and the second is that channels that connect to the bones can influence the eight extraordinary channels, jing, and source qi. The divergent channels connect to the superficial layers of the body, which include the skin and the bones, and their correspondences. Because the divergent channels connect to all these channels and substances, they can influence and treat them.

DISTAL NEEDLING

The *Ling Shu*, Chapter 7, "On Governing the Needles," presents the nine methods of needling. This chapter includes a way to treat different conditions. It emphasizes the importance of needling the correct channel system and depth. The practitioner should avoid pushing a pathogen deeper into the body. The practitioner should also be aware to needle at the superficial layer to treat superficial conditions, and to treat at the deep level to treat deeper-level conditions. Additionally, for conditions in the middle level, treat that level.

There are two especially interesting methods among the nine methods. The second method of the nine is "Needle the Distant Road." This method suggests *needling the lower part of the body to treat conditions of the upper part of the body*. The eighth method of the nine methods is "Opposite Needling." This method suggests treating the right side when the disease is on the left side, and treating the left side for conditions on the right side. These two methods guide the practitioner to use the lower body to treat the upper body, and to use one side of the body to treat the opposite side (contralateral needling). These methods are found in modern clinical applications of the divergent channels.

The same chapter also presents that there are three depths to acupuncture and provides the following guidance:

> Thus, the "rule of acupuncture" says, to begin, needle shallowly in order to expel the evil qi and to let the blood and qi come forward. Afterwards, needle deeply in order to affect the yin qi's evil. Finally, needle extremely deeply in order to descend to the valley qi.[21]

This quote expresses there are three levels of the body. Some practitioners call them the wei, ying, and yuan levels. The wei level includes the sinews, connecting, and divergent channels; the ying level includes the primary channels (the divergent channels connect to the organs); and the yuan level includes the eight extraordinary and divergent channels. A treatment strategy should include where the condition is located and target it with the corresponding channels. Because the divergent channels connect to the three levels, they can assist in treating conditions of all three levels. These relationships are unique to the divergent channels.

EMOTIONS AND THE DIVERGENT CHANNELS

The *Ling Shu*, Chapter 8, "The Roots of Spirit," presents the emotions and their relationships to the internal organs. The primary channels are extensions of the organs, so the conditions in the primary channels can influence the organs and the emotions. Stress from our lifestyle can influence the channels, the organs, and the emotions. The connecting channels (blood channels), which hold emotions, can transfer them to the organs. "The Roots of Spirit" shows how conditions, both internal and external, can influence spirit (mind) and our emotional condition. The divergent channels can assist in releasing the imbalanced emotional energy from the organs and channels.

RIVERS AND CHANNELS

The *Ling Shu*, Chapter 12, "Rivers and Channels," presents how the channels are images of water flows in our environment. This chapter matches large rivers from ancient China to the channels on the body. The pattern of the rivers (channels) is the exact distribution of the divergent channels, found in Chapter 11 of the *Ling Shu*.

This chapter also partitions the body into heaven and earth: heaven is above the waist and earth is below the waist. In some traditions, the confluent points are grouped as heaven and earth points. For example, for the Bladder and the Kidneys, Bladder 40, middle of the crook, is the earth point, and Bladder 10, tian zhu, celestial pillar, is the heaven point. The two points are often the first points needled to stimulate the divergent channels. Ideally, additional pathway points are included in the treatment.

THE MUSCLE CHANNELS

The *Ling Shu*, Chapter 13, "The Muscle Channels," presents the pathways and conditions of the muscle channels. The chapter also presents the type of conditions that can manifest during each of the twelve months of the year. Additionally, the painful (ashi) points are presented and suggested to be included in a treatment.

MEASUREMENTS IN REFERENCE TO THE BONES

The *Ling Shu*, Chapter 14, "Measurements in Reference to the Bones," lists a detailed explanation of the major bones of the body. The preceding chapter presents the muscle channels, which includes the tendons. The tendons connect to bones; they influence each other. Anatomically, tendons and bones are at the superficial layer, and they influence wei qi. Bones are also related to jing, source qi, and the eight extraordinary channels. Bones are a bridge to the exterior and interior, and the wei and yuan levels. The divergent channels can influence bones because they originate at the big bones and joints. They can influence the range of influence of bones. They can move vital substances to the exterior aspect of bones, as well as to the interior aspect of bones.

These relationships work to transfer pathogenic factors as well. The body can divert pathogens into these locations as a preventative action. If they are not treated they can cause chronic and more serious conditions. Clearing these areas is important for health and vitality. Qi Gong has many physical movements that clear the joints and muscles of pathogenic factors.

The great Han dynasty physician Hua Tuo is famous for saying: "The moving hinge collects no rust." Daily movement clears away pathogenic factors and allows a healthy circulation of qi and blood. The divergent channels can assist in this clearing of pathogenic factors, and in a healthy circulation of qi and blood.

NEEDLING TECHNIQUE METHODS

The *Ling Shu*, Chapter 1, "Of Nine Needles and Twelve Source Points, 'The Laws of Heaven,'" contains the basic needling strategies:

> The method of acupuncture is to tonify hollowness, disperse fullness, and dredge stasis. When these methods are applied, the pathogen will be weakened. Needling slow, then quick, produces tonification. Needling quick, then slow, produces reducing.[22]

The *Ling Shu* offers three major treatment strategies: reinforcing, reducing, and dredging. From an acupuncture viewpoint, reinforcing means guiding vital substances to an area. Reducing means guiding substances or pathogenic factors away from an area. And dredging means clearing stasis. All treatments should include one of these three actions.

There are three methods for reinforcing and reducing in the *Ling Shu*. The first method is based on the respiration of the patient, the second method is based on the insertion and withdrawal speed of the needle, and the third method is about how the point is covered with a cotton ball after the needle is removed.

The first reinforcing method is to insert the needle on the patient's exhalation and withdraw it on the patient's inhalation. The second reinforcing method is to insert the needle slowly and withdraw it quickly. And the third reinforcing method is to cover the hole immediately after the needle is withdrawn.

The first reducing method is to insert the needle on the patient's inhalation and withdraw it on the patient's exhalation. The second reducing method is to insert the needle quickly and withdraw it slowly. And the third reducing method is to wait before covering the hole after the needle is withdrawn.

Treatment strategies should include the following two plans: when there is a deficiency, apply the reinforcing method; and when there is excess, apply the reducing method. When there is a deficiency, the goal is to guide vital substances to an area or organ to reinforce. When there is excess, the goal is to reduce or guide the pathogenic factor away from an area and release it. These treatments and needling methods should be included in divergent channel treatments.

The *Su Wen* and the *Ling Shu* practitioners presented a variety of traditions and methods for practicing acupuncture. One main theory includes the energetics of Yin and Yang organs. Yin organs gather and store. Yang organs empty and release. Applying acupuncture based on the intrinsic nature of the organs includes reinforcing Yin organs when there is a deficiency, and reducing Yang organs when there is excess. Any one or a combination of the reinforcing methods presented can be applied. For example, if there is a Kidney deficiency, reinforce Kidney points. Reinforcing based on respiration, insertion, and covering the hole can be applied. When there is an excess of a Yang channel, for instance Stomach fire, reduce Stomach points. Reducing based on respiration, insertion, and whether to cover the hole can be applied.

These *Ling Shu* and *Su Wen* theories, principles, and applications can be applied to the divergent channels in clinical practice. It is my experience that including them in practice increases clinical effectiveness.

Part III
Clinical Applications

CHAPTER 10

THE CLINICAL APPLICATIONS OF DIVERGENT CHANNELS THEORY

The divergent channels are an essential part of acupuncture channel theory, and are very important in clinical practice. The divergent channels can directly treat conditions in their own channels; they can also support treating any of the other channel systems in the body.

The foundation needling methods of acupuncture should be applied to divergent channel treatments. The methods are to reinforce, reduce, or dredge. Generally, one of the following goals is applied.

The first goal is to guide vital substances to an area to reinforce an organ. The second goal is to reduce. This action guides pathogenic factors or vital substances outward, usually to the exterior. It releases pathogenic factors. The third goal is to increase circulation to clear stagnations.

The divergent channels assist in mobilizing the body's resources to reinforce, reduce, or dredge. They are energy fields (channels) that can influence other channels and the entire body. They can cause a reaction that permeates the channels they are connected to in the treatment.

The divergent channels are one of the most potent channel systems that link channels and areas of the body. This function of the divergent channels brings a clarity and focus as to how to utilize these channels in clinical practice.

THE CLINICAL ACUPUNCTURE FRAMEWORK

The *Ling Shu* discusses the body's system of channels and their pathways, at both the interior and exterior areas of the body. It goes to great lengths to emphasize the importance of knowing which channels are imbalanced. This includes symptoms, conditions, diseases, and pulses to identify the channels and organs that are imbalanced.

These qualities and correspondences are the body's messages about the condition of each organ and channel. Being clear about the channel and organ being treated is essential in an effective treatment. Equally important is the message we send to the body as practitioners. The order of the acupuncture channels and the points treated is key to the message sent to the body. The exact order of insertion of the needles in the body is a critical part of the message.

A goal when needling the divergent channels is to stimulate their channels, which causes a reaction along the pathways and their connections. It is this reaction that is the basis of why the divergent channels can assist in treating other channels and organs. The reaction has two main functions. The first reaction is within its own channel, and its Yin–Yang paired channel. The second is the reaction it has on the body, the vital substances, pathogenic factors, and the other channel systems in the treatment.

For example, if a patient had chronic anger, and he or she wanted to release this emotion and pattern, a Liver and Gallbladder divergent channel treatment could be applied. The luo channel and the luo points on the Liver and Gallbladder channels can be bled, or plum blossomed, which is an outlet to allow the anger to more easily be released from the body. A Gallbladder and Liver divergent channels treatment can assist in guiding the anger qi to the luo points and area to be released. Additionally, treating these channels influences the modality applied in the treatment. They can enhance the function of the modality. Modalities such as bloodletting, plum blossom, gua sha, and moxibustion can be included with divergent channel treatments.

A FRAMEWORK FOR DIVERGENT CHANNEL TREATMENT PLANS

Designing treatments for each person is the essence of Chinese medicine. A good way to approach designing divergent channel treatments is with a framework, including modules. After you make a diagnosis and select the channels to be treated, consider how to stimulate the entire channel(s). The following outline is a guide to developing divergent channel treatments:

1. Treat the confluent points. Begin with the lower and then treat the upper confluent points. This stimulates the channel and causes a reaction in the channels. It can be a reinforcement or reducing needling method.

    The confluent points are where the divergent channel's Yin–Yang pairs interact. By treating them we can stimulate both of the divergent paired channels, creating a synergetic effect. Stimulating the channels includes a movement, which can be up and down the channel, as well as to the interior and exterior (inside and outward). Generally, the movement of these channels will be one of these four directions. Acupuncture can enhance these movements.

    An alternative to the confluent points is treating the beginning and ending points. They can be used with the confluent points, or without them.

2. Select points along the divergent channels pathway. The points can be in the anatomical area of the condition. They can also be points with functions that treat the condition. They can also be points that stimulate the entire channel(s).

3. Select points with the same strategy in steps 1–2 for the divergent channel's Yin–Yang pair channel. For example, what is applied on the Spleen channel can be applied on the Stomach channel.

4. Select points from other channel systems that can treat the condition. For example, if there is an organ deficiency, include source, sea, mu, shu, and five-phase reinforcement points. Select from the wide range of acupuncture points in the channels.

5. Consider adding other healing modalities in the treatment. The combination of multiple applications increases clinical effectiveness. Moxibustion, tui na (body work), lancet, and plum blossom are effective methods to be included in divergent channel treatments.

Keys to using the divergent channels in clinical practice are the same as for any other acupuncture channel system. Learning the pathways, and the points along the pathways, is essential to clinical effectiveness. Including the needling technique in the treatment is one of the most important contributors to clinical effectiveness. An important element of a treatment is the exact order in which the channels and the points are treated. Plan which channels you want to treat first, and then plan the exact order the needles will be inserted. The order creates a powerful healing synergy.

THE DIVERGENT CHANNELS AND THE CHANNEL SYSTEM

The divergent channels can be used with all the channel systems. Examples of how to use the divergent channels with each of the main channel systems are now presented. Use these examples as a guide for creating your own treatments.

Method 1: Treating the divergent channels pathways

The first method is to treat conditions in the divergent channels pathways. In a macro view, all the pathologies and imbalances of the body have the potential to move into the divergent channels. Each treatment begins with diagnosis and a treatment plan. The treatment plan will include reinforcing, reducing, or dredging. An example for treating the pathways of the divergent channels is when there is bi syndrome (wind-damp-cold) on the spine, from Thoracic Vertebra 11 to Lumbar Vertebra 4. The treatment is to resolve and clear the bi syndrome. A treatment plan can be to reduce the Bladder and Kidneys' divergent channels. These channels flow along the spine. The goal is to create an energetic flow that moves the bi syndrome from the spine, and the Bladder and Kidneys' divergent channels, and then out of the body.

Method 2: Supporting the internal organs and the primary channels

When there is a diagnosis of an internal organ deficiency, the divergent channels can be treated to assist in reinforcing the organ. For example, if there is Spleen qi deficiency, the goal is to reinforce the Spleen. A strategy can be to select points on the Spleen and Stomach primary channel. The Spleen and Stomach divergent channels can be used to assist in the reinforcing movement. Reinforcing the Spleen and Stomach divergent channels creates a momentum that guides qi to the Spleen, to reinforce it.

If there is a condition of Stomach fire, the Spleen and Stomach divergent channels could be reduced to assist in releasing and clearing the Stomach fire.

Method 3: Supporting the muscle channels

When a patient has back pain, for example pain along the para-spinal muscles, the Bladder and Kidney divergent channels can assist in the treatment. If there is bi syndrome, these channels could assist in clearing the bi syndrome, as well as circulating qi and blood to clear the channels and area. There are points on these channels that a practitioner may select in their standard treatment for back pain, for example Bladder 40, Bladder 10, and the Hua Tuo Jia Ji points. A difference between needling a point or two from the channel, and a combination of points on the divergent channels, is the ability to stimulate the entire channel, and not just an area. A divergent channels treatment can assist in relaxing the muscles, move qi and blood, and create an outward movement or force to move the bi syndrome pathogenic factor(s) to the surface to be released. A standard muscle (sinew) channel treatment can include superficial needling to stimulate the wei qi, which can release the pathogenic factor. Cupping, gua sha, plum blossom, and liniments can assist in the releasing function.

Method 4: Supporting the connecting channels

The classical application of the connecting channels is to treat blood conditions and emotions. The divergent channels can support the connecting channels when treating these conditions. They are especially effective in treating emotional conditions. For instance, if a person has repressed Liver qi and a hun imbalance, plum blossoming the Liver and Gallbladder connecting points Liver 5 and Gallbladder 37 is very effective. Applying a Liver and Gallbladder divergent channel treatment is very effective in bringing the emotional energy to the surface. The connecting channel treatment allows the release of the emotional qi. Plum blossoming is a gentle way to create the outlet for the release. Classically, blood letting with a lancet would be applied on the channel and points. The divergent channels can assist in treating acute or chronic emotional conditions.

Method 5: Supporting the eight extraordinary channels

The divergent channels can assist the eight extraordinary channels to support other channel systems. For example, if a patient has chronic fatigue with Kidney Yang deficiency, a Du channel treatment may be selected to reinforce the Kidneys. A Bladder and Kidney divergent channels treatment can support that treatment plan. It can help guide the vital substances from the Du channel to the Kidneys. Combining these channels creates a very effective treatment.

The divergent channels are a major part of the acupuncture system. Including them in your acupuncture treatments can increase clinical effectiveness.

CASE STUDIES

The following case studies are presented as examples of how to apply the divergent channels in clinical practice. The essence of Chinese medicine is making a unique diagnosis for each person, and then creating a unique treatment plan. The cases presented are guides for learning to create divergent channel treatments. The cases contain a framework or an approach to clinical applications.

Case 1

A 54-year-old male is suffering from back pain. The pain ranges from Thoracic Vertebra 11 to Lumbar Vertebra 4.

DIAGNOSIS

Bi syndrome (wind-damp-cold). The Western medical diagnosis is arthritis.

TREATMENT PLAN

The treatment is to resolve the bi syndrome by reducing the area in which the bi syndrome is located. The Bladder and Kidneys divergent channels pathways flow along the spine. These channels will be used to assist in clearing the bi syndrome.

The bi syndrome is also influencing the muscle channels (sinew channels) adjacent to the spine. The treatment plan will include clearing the bi syndrome from the muscle channels, and relaxing the muscle channels and the local muscles.

TREATMENT STRATEGY

1. Release the Bladder muscle channels.

2. Release the Bladder and Kidneys divergent channels.

3. Select acupuncture points to treat the local pain.

4. Select acupuncture points to treat the bi syndrome.

5. Promote urination to assist in releasing the wind-damp-cold.

    a. Needle Bladder 40, Bladder 10, Du 20, Bladder 10 and Bladder 40.

    b. Needle Du 16 and Du 6.

    c. Needle Hua Tuo Jia Ji points at ashi locations.

    d. Needle Small Intestine 3 and Bladder 65.

    e. Needle Bladder 11.

    f. Apply moxibustion.

    g. Treat Bladder 64 and Bladder 28, the source and back shu points of the Bladder, to promote urination.

Treatment modalities

1. Perform tui na or a form of massage on the local area (the Bladder muscle channels).

2. Perform a reducing method of acupuncture on the Bladder and Kidney divergent channels: a, b, c.

3. Needle the stream points on the Hand and Foot Tai Yang channels, and the influential point of bone (Bladder 11): d, e. These treat bi syndrome and pain.

4. Apply moxibustion on local areas of bi syndrome (pain) that enhance the treatment: f. Moxibustion is one of the best modalities for treating pain.

5. Perform acupuncture on points to promote urination: g.

Case 2

A 32-year-old female has suffered from anger and frustration for ten years. She wants to address this condition. She is in therapy with a psychologist.

DIAGNOSIS

Liver qi stagnation with repressed anger. The hun spirit is repressed.

TREATMENT PLAN

Release the anger and frustration, and soothe Liver qi stagnation.

TREATMENT STRATEGY

Release the Liver and Gallbladder divergent channels to assist in releasing the repressed anger and hun spirit.

Treat the Liver connecting channels to release anger, frustration, and the Liver qi stagnation.

TREATMENT MODALITIES

1. Perform plum blossom on Right Liver 5 and Left Gallbladder 37. These are the connecting (luo) points of the Liver and Gallbladder. Classically, these points are bled to release the emotional energy stored in the blood.

2. Apply a Liver and Gallbladder divergent channel treatment.

3. Suggest the patient walk each day. Walking taxes the tendons, and the Liver and Gallbladder. Walking is a gentle, natural way to reduce the Liver and Gallbladder imbalances (anger, frustration, and a repressed hun spirit).

The divergent channel treatment includes Ren 2, Gallbladder 1, Du 20, Gallbladder 1, and Ren 2 again. Then treat Liver 14; this is on the divergent pathway, and is the mu point of the Liver.

San Jiao channel points are included to assist in releasing the pathogenic factors: San Jiao 6, Gallbladder 41.

TREATMENT PLAN DETAIL

1. Perform the luo treatment.

2. Treat the divergent channel. Apply the reducing method on Ren 2, Left Gallbladder 1, Du 20, and Right Gallbladder 1, and re-stimulate Ren 2. Reduce Liver 14.

3. Reduce San Jiao 6. This point stimulates the three jiao and can guide the treatment outward. It is the horary point. Gallbladder 41 is the stream and horary point (wood point on the wood channel). It is also the opening point of the Dai channel. It is a major Shao Yang point. It has a powerful effect on releasing. Both points are on Shao Yang channels, and they can create a strong energetic force to release. These two points support the releasing treatment plan.

Case 3

A 46-year-old male has chronic fatigue. He complains of gas and bloating after eating meals.

DIAGNOSIS

Spleen and Stomach qi deficiency.

TREATMENT PLAN

Reinforce the Spleen and Stomach.

Treatment strategy

1. Reinforce the Spleen and Stomach divergent channels to support the Spleen and Stomach primary channels and the internal organs.

2. Reinforce the Spleen and Stomach primary channels.

Treatment modalities

The divergent channels treatment should be inserted in this exact order: Left Stomach 30, Left Stomach 1, Du 20, Right Stomach 1, Right Stomach 30. Stomach 30 and Stomach 1 are the confluent points. Du 20 is used to assist in moving the treatment from one side of the body to the other, increasing the energetic influence on the divergent channels. Du 20 also reinforces the Spleen, and strengthens its ability to ascend gu qi to the Lungs.

Ren 12 is on the Stomach divergent channel pathway. It is also the front mu of the Stomach, and it reinforces the Stomach and Spleen.

The Spleen and Stomach primary channels treatment is Spleen 3 and Stomach 36. These are the source and the sea points. They both powerfully reinforce the Stomach (Stomach 36 is also the lower he sea, the earth, and the horary point). Stomach 30 and Stomach 36 are also the sea of grain points; they powerfully reinforce the Stomach and Spleen.

Case 4

A 58-year-old female has experienced insomnia for 20 years. She has difficulty falling asleep. She does not fall asleep until 1 am or later. She has tried natural remedies with little success.

Diagnosis

Heart fire.

Treatment plan
Clear Heart fire.

Treatment strategy

1. Clear heat from the Heart and the Heart primary channel with the Heart and Small Intestine divergent channels.

2. Perform plum blossom on Small Intestine 7. This is the connecting point of the Small Intestine connecting channel. Plum blossom allows the Heart fire to be released from the body.

Treatment modalities

The divergent channels treatment is right Gallbladder 22, right Bladder 1, left Bladder 1, and left Gallbladder 22. These are the divergent channels' confluent points. Ren 17 and Stomach 12, which are on the divergent channels pathways, are included in the treatment.

Reduce Ren 17. Gua sha Stomach 12: this allows heat to be released from the Heart and the Small Intestine channels and organs.

Plum blossom Small Intestine 7 bilaterally. This is the luo point of the Small Intestine, and it is the Yin–Yang channel of the Heart channel. The luo points can release heat from the channels.

Case 5

A 56-year-old woman states that she has difficulty taking responsibility for her actions in relationships with other people. She continually blames others for any challenges and difficulties that occur in her life.

Diagnosis
Pericardium deficiency.

Treatment plan

Reinforce the Pericardium and the San Jiao divergent channels. The treatment also includes reinforcing the zhi (the Kidneys and willpower). The zhi and the Kidneys contain our will. Reinforcing the Kidneys, the zhi, and the will can allow the person to have the willpower to take responsibility for their actions.

Treatment strategy

The divergent channels treatment begins with the confluent points of the Pericardium and the San Jiao. The points are Ren 12 and San Jiao 16. These points assist in stimulating the divergent channels to reinforce the Pericardium.

After the divergent channels points are treated, needle Pericardium 7; this is the source point of the Pericardium channel. Pericardium 7 reinforces the Pericardium. Reinforcing the Pericardium increases the ability to respond to life interactions with integrity.

Treatment modalities

Kidney 3 and Ren 6 are needled to reinforce the Kidneys and the zhi. These are the source point of the Kidneys, and the sea of qi. They are major points to reinforce the Kidneys and essence. The treatment can reinforce the Pericardium and the Kidneys. As the Heart protector, the Pericardium has a relationship with the Kidneys in a similar way as the Heart. The Kidneys and the Heart are Shao Yin; the Pericardium can be viewed as part of that energetic connection.

Consider including the Yin Wei channel. Because this is a chronic condition, the eight extraordinary channels can be added to this treatment and the Yin Wei channel could support this. It can help release this woman from her chronic patterns of behavior and conditioning. A Yin Wei treatment could be Kidney 9, Spleen 16, and Liver 14. Insert the needles on the right side first, and apply the reducing method to begin the process of releasing. Begin the treatment with the Yin Wei channel and then treat the Pericardium and San Jiao divergent channels, and then treat the primary channels.

Case 6

A 61-year-old female has severe sadness, depression, and grief from the loss of her husband five years ago. She has no history of unusual emotional conditions. She has a difficult time expressing these feelings about the loss of her husband to others; rather, she has internalized them (suppressed them). She has been in therapy for six months, and feels it has helped. She wants to be able to express the emotions and begin the process of moving forward in her life.

Diagnosis

Sadness, depression, and grief from the loss of her husband. It is a po disharmony (the Lung's shen).

Treatment plan

Release the emotions in the Lung and Large Intestine channel system (the connecting and primary channels).

Treatment strategy

Perform a luo and divergent channels treatment, as well as using the horary and window of the sky point on the Lung channel.

Treatment modalities

The treatment has three parts. They would be applied in the exact order listed:

1. Plum blossom right Lung 7 and left Large Intestine 6. These are the connecting points (luo points) of the Lungs and the Large Intestine channels, and they influence the po. The Lung is a Yin channel and corresponds to the right side, and the Large Intestine is a Yang channel and corresponds to the left side. Treat the matched polarity of the points and channels. Plum blossoming allows the imbalanced energy (emotion) to be released.

2. Perform a releasing (clearing) divergent treatment on the Lung and Large Intestine divergent channels points. This stimulates the divergent channels to move the emotional energy outward. Begin with Stomach 12 and Large Intestine 18. These are the confluent points. These points assist in stimulating the divergent channels.

   Perform a reducing needling technique on the following divergent channels points to assist in releasing the emotional energy in the Lungs, and the Large Intestine channel system: Lung 1, Large Intestine 15, and Gallbladder 21. These points when combined with the confluent points assist in releasing the emotional energy in the luo channels and the Lung organ. The five Yin organs house the five shen, and the Lungs house the po shen.

3. Complete the treatment by needling Lung 8 and Lung 3. Lung 8 is the channel ditch, and it is the horary point (the metal point on the metal channel). Reducing this point draws the imbalanced energy out from the ditch in the channel. It assists in releasing the sadness, depression, and grief from the Lung channel system. Lung 3 is a window of the sky point, and assists in releasing the po emotional energy from the body.

Key to applying the divergent channels in clinical practice is having clarity of the area and the points along the pathways. Strategically selecting points and areas to treat is both an art and a science. Table 10.1 summarizes the main points along the divergent channels. Refer to this chart when considering points for a divergent channels treatment.

Table 10.1 The divergent channels confluent and pathway points

Channel	Confluent points	Divergent channel pathway points
Bladder	Bladder 40	Bladder 40, 36, 32, 15, 44, 10 Du 1, Du 4, Du 11, Hua Tuo Jia Ji points Ren 3, Ren 4
Kidneys	Bladder 10	Kidney 10, Bladder 40, Du 4, Bladder 23, Bladder 52, Bladder 10 Gallbladder 26, Spleen 15, Kidney 16, Ren 8
Gallbladder	Gallbladder 30 or Ren 2	Ren 2, Ren 3, Liver 13, Gallbladder 24, Gallbladder 25, Liver 14, Ren 14, Stomach 12, Ren 23, Stomach 5, Ren 24 Gallbladder 30, Gallbladder 1
Liver	Gallbladder 1	Liver 5, Ren 2, Gallbladder 1
Stomach	Stomach 30	Stomach 30, Ren 12, Ren 17, Ren 22, Ren 23, Stomach 9, Stomach 4, Bladder 1
Spleen	Bladder 1 Large Intestine 20 Stomach 1	Spleen 12, Stomach 30, Stomach 9, Ren 23, Bladder 1
Small Intestine	Bladder 1	Small Intestine 10, Heart 1, Gallbladder 22, Ren 14, Ren 17, Stomach 12, Small Intestine 18, Bladder 1
Heart	Gallbladder 22	Heart 1, Gallbladder 22, Ren 17, Ren 23, Bladder 1
San Jiao	Ren 12	Du 20, San Jiao 16, Stomach 12, Ren 17, Ren 12
Pericardium	San Jiao 16 Gallbladder 12 San Jiao 19	Pericardium 1, Ren 17, Ren 12, Ren 23, San Jiao 16
Large Intestine	Stomach 12	Large Intestine 15, Stomach 12, Large Intestine 18, Stomach 15 Du 14, Gallbladder 21
Lungs	Large Intestine 18	Lung 1, Gallbladder 22, Stomach 12, Large Intestine 18

Part IV
NEI DAN INNER MEDITATION

CHAPTER 11

INTRODUCTION TO NEI DAN INNER MEDITATION

The ancient Chinese perceived the inseparable relationship between nature and humanity. Understanding the universe was a central theme for them, and the relationship between humanity and the forces of the universe was a predominant focus. These ancient people created a variety of ways to communicate their insights, which included diagrams, models, and theories to explain the universe around them. During this time the healers were called the *Wu*, who would become masters of the formula. They developed formulas to communicate with the forces of nature and supernatural beings (such as the *eight immortals*). These people were also called *fangshi* (*fang-shih*), which means masters of the method/masters of the formula. The formulas would expand to other areas of life, including herbs, acupuncture, and nei dan (inner meditation). In ancient China, adepts called internal alchemists developed formulas for spiritual development and self-realization. In this case the formulas were meditations. These include many of the theories, principles, and cosmic relationships found in the *Su Wen* and the *Ling Shu*. The five phases are a major aspect of these inner meditations (nei dan).

The *Ling Shu* is the Han dynasty classic on acupuncture. "Ling Shu" can be translated as the "spiritual axis" or the "spiritual compass." As a compass, it can identify a current location and reveal the way to a destination. This classic book presents a model for understanding existing health conditions, as well as offering directions and guidance to find health, longevity, and spiritual realization. Chapter 54 of the *Ling Shu*, "The Allotted Year of a Human's Life," offers advice on the meaning of spirit (shen). Qi Bo states: "When one's blood and energy are complete and harmonized, when nourishing and protective Qi are complete and penetrating, when the five viscera are complete and matured, the spirit qi is sheltered in the Heart and mind, and the animal spirit and human soul complete the organs, the person is complete."

Blood, nourishing qi, and the animal spirit are Yin. Qi, wei qi, and the human soul are Yang. The Heart and mind are Yang, and the organs are Yin. A meaning of this description of spirit is: when Yin and Yang are in harmony, vital substances, organs, and emotions are in harmony, and the body and spirit are unified. This unification can lead to an insight. When we are in balance and harmony within ourselves and with the world around us, our body and spirit naturally unify and we become a living expression of spirit. It is my understanding that this explanation mirrors the diamond-in-the-rough insight presented in this book. Harmonizing the Yin and Yang will clear the rough. When the rough is cleared, the diamond, which is spirit, is revealed.

Chapter 7 of this book presents important five shen relationships within the body. These relationships comprise a large part of the inner meditation called "Fusion of the Five Phases." I also call this meditation *Five Shen Nei Dan*. The Taoist hermit One Cloud traveled throughout China and learned internal alchemy/nei dan during his travels. He taught the Fusion of the Five Phases nei dan to Mantak Chia. I learned this nei dan in 1984, and have practiced and taught it ever since. While studying the *Su Wen* and *Ling Shu* I saw that many parts of the formula were in those classic medical texts. I have slightly modified the formula based on my practice of this meditation, and my medical knowledge. Five Shen Nei Dan is a profound meditation to transform emotions. It transforms emotional qi into vitality. This cultivation can clear "the rough in our life"; it begins the process of attuning to spirit and self-realization. A primary objective of this cultivation is to realize that our emotions are just one aspect of our life, and not the most essential one. When the emotions (and stresses) are in balance, the spirit will appear. This nei dan assists in finding this balance and spirit realization by way of self-cultivation.

This inner meditation begins with a deep understanding of the five organs—the Heart, Lungs, Liver, Spleen, and Kidneys—and their correspondences. The meditation works with the qi, elements, colors, temperatures, and emotions that correspond to the five internal organs. Balance is the key principle in Chinese philosophy, medicine, and health: balancing the five organs is essential for health and vitality.

China is one of the most diverse cultures in the world. This diversity includes many spiritual traditions. Four great traditions exist in China: indigenous culture, Taoism, Confucianism, and Buddhism. There are many branches within each of these traditions, and there are also a variety of combinations of these traditions. It would be virtually impossible to say that there is one view of any of the traditions. In my experience, we need to obtain clarity on certain aspects within these traditions in order to be able to use them in clinical practice. There are three insights within these traditions that provide a framework for clinical applications, as well as for personal development. The first such insight is *original spirit*, the second insight is *a diamond in the rough*, and the third is the *five shen*. These insights are now presented briefly; the five shen are also discussed in various places throughout this book.

INSIGHTS
Yuan shen (original spirit)

Chinese culture contains a variety of spiritual traditions. Each of these traditions includes insights that form the basis of its teachings and practices. One insight is that each person has a *yuan shen* (original spirit), and this spirit is part of the universal spirit. What this means is that the creator and creation are one. They are an undivided whole. By experiencing one's yuan shen, the unity of life is realized; the inseparable nature of life is realized; and the clarity of one's true nature is realized. By directly experiencing one's yuan shen, it also becomes clear what yuan shen is not. This insight is essential to self-realization, health, happiness, and transformation. Acupuncture can have a profound influence on releasing attachments and imprints that prevent an individual from realizing their yuan shen.

A diamond in the rough

A diamond in the rough is an image that illustrates how the process of self-realization can occur. Each person has a diamond. The diamond is the yuan shen. The rough includes the stresses, conditioning, imprints, patterns, emotions, and unfavorable influences that exist in our life. We all have a diamond shining within, and we all have rough. The amount and types of rough vary among people. Acupuncture can assist in releasing, clearing, and removing the rough, thereby allowing insight and alignment with the diamond. This process can be life-changing, and can provide additional inspiration and motivation for further changes. It can inspire a person to live in a way that allows synchronization with shen (becoming aware of it)—a living expression of shen.

The five shen

Chinese medicine includes a unique understanding of the psychological and spiritual aspects of a person's life. Chapter 5 of the *Su Wen*, "The Manifestation of Yin and Yang from the Macrocosm to the Microcosm," presents the *five shen*. These shen are a model for understanding patterns of disharmony. The five shen are the *shen, yi, po, zhi,* and *hun*; they relate to the Heart, Spleen, Lungs, Kidneys, and Liver. Shen is Yang, and the five organs are Yin. The ancients viewed the Yin organs as housing the shen; Yang must have a Yin to contain it. The conditions of the shen can influence the Yin organs, and conversely the conditions of the Yin organs can influence the shen. The shen relate to the five Yin organs and their correspondences.

Each shen has specific psychological qualities. These are matched to their corresponding organ and channel. This provides a way to identify which organ and associated channel system is imbalanced and consequentially should be treated. Nei dan and Qi Gong traditions offer many insights into the five shen. This section of the book presents some of these important insights.

Each of the five shen has unique corresponding emotions (qualities) that reflect their underlying condition, the key ones of which are:

- Hastiness, impatience, arrogance, cruelty, and hatred correspond to the Heart *shen*. Joy and love are the natural virtues.

- Worry, repetitive thinking, obsessive behavior, and jealousy correspond to the Spleen *yi*. Openness is the natural virtue.

- Sadness, depression, loneliness, isolation, and the inability to forgive correspond to the Lung *po*. Courage and righteousness are the natural virtues.

- Fear corresponds to the Kidney *zhi*, and gentleness is the natural virtue.

- Anger, irritability, and frustration correspond to the Liver *hun*, and kindness is the natural virtue.

When these emotions are imbalanced, by matching the emotion of the corresponding shen to its associated organ, one can use this as the basis for cultivation and treatment. In the model of the diamond in the rough, imbalances of these emotions are "the rough." Acupuncture and nei dan can assist in clearing the roughness, revealing the shining light of the diamond (i.e., the yuan shen). Nei dan releases chronic/old patterns of roughness, and redirects a person to their diamond. Union with your yuan shen can inspire, motivate, and provide the impetus for change and transformation.

THE THREE DAN TIAN

There are many Qi Gong and nei dan traditions. Most of the traditions include the three dan tian in their theory and practice. The three dan tian are three areas in the body (Figure 11.1). These areas are sometimes called jiao, burners, or centers. Dan tian means "energy field." It is an area, not a specific point. Each dan tian has organs located in it. Moreover, each dan tian contains and influences different types of vital substances (such as types of qi). Understanding the functions of each dan tian allows for identifying imbalances of organs, vital substances, and emotional conditions.

178 THE DIVERGENT CHANNELS—JING BIE

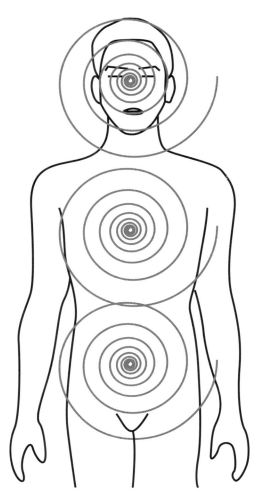

Figure 11.1 The three dan tian

The lower dan tian ranges from the perineum (the area around the anus) to the coccyx, and up the spine to the Kidneys, where it flows across to the umbilicus, and then back down to the perineum. The lower dan tian includes the Kidneys, adrenals, Bladder, sexual organs, pubic bone, pelvis, coccyx, sacrum, and lumbar. This dan tian influences the processes of the gate of vitality. It is the ming men cooking jing, creating source qi (steam). The Kidneys store jing and the gate of vitality. There are two Kidneys: one is Kidney Yang and the other is Kidney Yin. They are the foundation Yin and Yang of the entire body. The Kidneys provide these substances to all other organs. The quality of the Kidneys influences all organs and the entire body.

The middle dan tian ranges from the area above the lower dan tian to the area of the neck. This dan tian includes two energetic influences. The first influence relates to the Spleen and the Stomach. The second influence relates to the Lungs and the Heart. Regarding the first influence, the Spleen and Stomach are the earth element. The elements and functions of these two organs represent post-natal influences. On a physical level, they include the ability to transform food and drink into energy. On a psycho-emotional level, they correspond to the yi spirit and include the consequences of our actions.

One way to change unfavorable post-natal influences related to the physical body is to change one's diet and exercise. On a psycho-emotional level, the yi digests, processes, and organizes our experiences in life. From this comes our understanding of life and our ability to let go of experiences and emotions we do not need. It is essential to mature and refine our yi so that we may transform the imbalances that are created in this dan tian. In Chinese medicine, the Spleen holds blood in the vessels, and emotions are stored in the blood. Thus, the Spleen holds both blood and emotions. When the yi is imbalanced, the Spleen holds emotions that should be let go. This holding creates attachments to emotions, beliefs, and experiences, which may create further imbalances. Through nei dan cultivation, we may resolve imbalances created by the Spleen, Stomach, and the yi.

The second influence of the middle dan tian relates to the Lungs and the Heart. This area reflects the influences from society: the conditioning of culture and/or peer pressure. These influences can create imbalances. If they do, we need to cultivate this area, to release these imbalances and retain balance. This dan tian includes the po of the Lungs and the shen of the Heart.

The upper dan tian ranges from the neck to the top of the head (the crown). The lower dan tian represents earth, the middle dan tian represents humanity, and the upper dan tian represents heaven. The upper dan tian represents our connection to our yuan shen/original spirit (heaven). By transforming the lower and middle dan tian, we are ready to connect to our spirit. When we connect to our spirit, we are connected to the Tao. Imbalances in the lower and middle dan tian can create the illusion that this connection does not exist. Nei dan is one way to assist people in their self-realization of their spiritual nature.

Jing is our pre-natal essence and creates yuan qi/source qi. It also contains our genes and ancestral influences. The ability of the lower dan tian to function properly is essential for the Kidneys' ability to generate source qi. Nutrition, exercise, and a healthy lifestyle have a favorable effect on the Kidneys and their functioning. Stress, lack of exercise, poor diet, and excess sexual activity can drain jing, and weaken the Kidneys. A major aspect in obtaining health, vitality, and longevity is to live a lifestyle that supports the Kidneys, one that will support our foundation. Nei dan directly influences the functions of the lower dan tian and the Kidneys.

Taoist philosophy is earth-based. It contains a deep connection to earth and water. This connection includes the energetics, as well as the functions and movements of both earth and water. Water is the element of highest abundance on our planet, and it is likewise so in our body. The Chinese include water in their explanation of Chinese medicine. The observation of the flow of seas, rivers, streams, springs, and wells revealed how their country was nourished with water. Smooth flows of water brought bountiful harvests to agriculture, and life to humanity. Excesses, stagnations, blockages, and deficiencies in water flow caused flooding, drought, decay, and illness. The distribution of water throughout the country was seen as a model to be applied to the human body. Ancient healers viewed the flow of vital substances in the body as a mirror of the flow of water throughout a country. Since efficient water flow is essential for bountiful harvest, and since the drinking of water is essential for life, the flow of vital substances throughout the body is essential to health. Stagnations, deficiencies, or abnormal flows of vital substances cause illness. This circulatory model is fundamental to the function of the body. In nei dan, we implement this imagery of water circulation.

Chinese medicine includes descriptions of circulation patterns of vital substances. The acupuncture channel system is a pathway for their circulation. The terrain covered by the channels is the landscape. The channels include the sinew, luo, primary, divergent, and eight extraordinary channels. There are Qi Gong forms that influence each of these channels.

In Qi Gong and nei dan, there is an important principle: where the mind or intention goes, qi will follow. Wherever we move our intention or focus, qi will follow. Mind guides qi. In the Five Shen Nei Dan, we move our intention through the organs and channels as a means to clear, vitalize, and rejuvenate them. As these organs, channels, and qi are refined, we are able to move from "heavy energy" to "light energy." We are converting jing to shen. This is transformation.

Life is comprised of variations of qi. Qi can be dense or subtle: qi in dense form is jing; qi in subtle form is shen. Each variation of qi contains a vibration or frequency. Each of the three dan tian contains organs that produce a unique qi in its area. However, nei dan's viewpoint of the three dan tian is slightly different from the Chinese medical viewpoint. The Chinese medical view can be summarized as the following:

- The lower dan tian includes the Kidneys, and they produce yuan qi (source qi).

- The middle dan tian contains the Spleen and Stomach, and they produce gu qi (nutritive qi).

- The upper dan tian contains the Lungs and Heart, and they produce zong qi (gathering qi).

The three types of qi support the unfolding of jing to shen. The qi part of jing–qi–shen comprises each of the three treasures, and is the force guiding their unfolding from dense to subtle, or from jing to shen. One definition of alchemy might be: "Alchemy is making a conscious effort to change." Nei dan is a formula for change. The type of change that occurs is a shift from one's current state to a state of alignment with shen. A quest in our life is to seek and realize our spirit, and to live from it.

Nei dan begins by relaxing. Only by relaxing can the body begin to let go of stress and allow the normal circulation of vital substances throughout the body. This normal circulation begins the process of clearing imbalances. It is also energizing and rejuvenating to the body, mind, and spirit.

CHAPTER 12

THE CAULDRON

A cauldron is a large pot (kettle) that is used for cooking. Nei dan (alchemy) is a type of cooking. When cooking food there is a synergy that occurs in the cauldron. The food and fluids are cooked, thereby creating something new. The result is the integration of the cauldron, food, fluids, and heat/fire. Similar to this physical cauldron, we have an energetic cauldron in nei dan inner meditation. The energies of the organs and their correspondences are mixed and transformed in this cauldron, which is located in the solar plexus area. This area is the middle center (middle jiao) in this nei dan practice. (The original practice uses a cauldron (the yellow collection point) in the lower dan tian. If you feel the emotions are not being transformed effectively enough, try placing the yellow collection point in the lower dan tian.) The energies of the organs are brought into this cauldron to be mixed, integrated, and transformed. This is the Fusion of the Five Phases (five correspondences). These energies are transformed to original qi (yuan qi), which is the life force that can rejuvenate the body.

In Chinese medicine, the first energy in the body is called original qi. This qi will transform into the qi of the organs, the glands, the bones, the tendons, the blood, the brain, and the entire body. It is the life force that is derived from jing, and is the basis of the body, mind, and spirit. Each of the organs has its own qi: for example, Kidney qi, Liver qi, Heart qi, Spleen qi, and Lung qi. When the original qi flows into the organs, the nature of the original qi changes to the nature of the organs. The original qi is the most neutral qi. It can take the shape, form, and quality of the different parts of the body.

Say, for example, we try to relive a past experience or perhaps we have some experience that is very impactful on our life. Then part of our life force (qi) transforms into that experience or emotion. Consequently, we have the capacity to change our life force, whether favorably or unfavorably. In nei dan, we seek to change or transform our life force to its original qi. This allows the natural virtues of the organs to materialize.

The cauldron for the nei dan of emotional work is located in the middle of the body. This middle center is also called the middle jiao. In general, the lower center is behind and below the navel; the middle center is behind the solar plexus; and the upper center is behind the Heart center. The lower center corresponds to the Kidneys; the middle center corresponds to the Spleen; and the upper center corresponds to the Lungs and the Heart. The Spleen is the earth phase, which is the transformation phase. The earth phase can transform the other phases into their natural qi. In nei dan, we seek to transform imbalanced qi into balanced qi, and then subsequently into original qi. This original qi is then guided into the organs, the acupuncture channels, and then throughout the entire body. As a result of this circulation, the body can be healed and rejuvenated. Fusion of the Five Phases is a profound inner cultivation that transforms emotions and five-phase imbalances into vitality. This cultivation assists in harmonizing the emotional body, and allows awareness of the energy and spirit body.

NEI DAN PREPARATION: RELAXING WITH THE INNER SMILE MEDITATION

A wonderful way to begin a nei dan practice is with the inner smile meditation. This meditation generates a relaxing energy and can be practiced before the small heavenly orbit (microcosmic orbit; see the next chapter):

- Begin by sitting on a chair or on the floor. Your spine should be straight. Place the tip of your tongue at your palate (the roof of the mouth).

- Hold your hands in your lap in any way that is comfortable for you.

- Begin by smiling for a few minutes. When you feel relaxed, continue to smile, and place your mind's attention at the top of your head. Continue to smile throughout the entire meditation.

- Smile as you move your attention down the front and back of your head, and continue down to your neck.

- Continue smiling down your neck to your chest, and then down to the groin, and down the back to the lumbar area. Continue moving down your legs to your toes. Continue to smile throughout the meditation.

- Gently move your attention to your shoulders and smile down your arms. Take as much time as you need until you feel relaxed with a smiling energy.

- Gently bring your attention to the Heart center (between your nipples, behind the sternum). Smile into the Heart center and repeat the words "smiling, loving energy." Continue at the Heart center until you feel energy. This part of the meditation may last a few minutes.

- When you feel the smiling, loving energy at the Heart center, move your attention to your Heart. Repeat the words "joy" and "love." Feel joy and love in your Heart. Do this for one to five minutes, or until you feel joy and love.

- When you feel joy and love in your Heart, move your attention to your Lungs. Smile and repeat the word "courage." Feel courage in your Lungs. Do this until you feel energy in your Lungs.

- When you feel energy in your Lungs, move your attention to your Liver. Smile and repeat the word "kindness." Feel kindness in your Liver. Do this until you feel energy in your Liver.

- When you feel energy in your Liver, move your attention to your Spleen. Smile and repeat the word "openness." Feel openness in your Spleen. Do this until you feel energy in your Spleen.

- When you feel energy in your Spleen, move your attention to your Kidneys. Smile and repeat the word "gentleness." Feel gentleness in your Kidneys. Do this until you feel energy in your Kidneys.

Finish this meditation by gently moving your attention to the center of the lower dan tian (behind and below the navel). Focus there for three to five minutes. After completing the meditation, open your eyes, stretch, and enjoy. If you are going to continue with more nei dan practice, gently move on to the small heavenly orbit (microcosmic orbit), which is described in the next chapter.

CHAPTER 13

THE SMALL HEAVENLY ORBIT

The small heavenly orbit is comprised of the Ren and Du channels. The channels flow up the back of the body, and then down the front of the body. This circuit has a few names, such as the "heavenly orbit," the "small heavenly orbit," the "orbit," and the "microcosmic orbit." The Chinese name is *Xiao Zhou Tien*.

Nei dan inner meditation practice includes the Ren and Du channels. Lifestyle, poor diet, poor posture, and emotional imbalances can cause blockages in this orbit. By practicing nei dan, we can clear, cleanse, and energize these core channels. The efficiency of the functioning of the Ren and Du channels creates a direct influence on all the Yin–Yang correspondences in the body.

LOWER DAN TIAN

Life begins in the lower dan tian (Figure 13.1). Therefore, we begin nei dan in the lower dan tian. This dan tian is the center of the body. It is the root and the foundation. The lower dan tian is often called the *sea of qi*. It is the origin of source qi. It is the origin of Kidney Yin and Kidney Yang. These vital substances ignite, fuel, and vitalize the entire body. We begin our practice by focusing our attention in the sea of qi. Wherever we focus our attention, qi moves to that area. The yi has the ability to focus and concentrate. In Qi Gong theory, "focusing attention" is under the control of the Spleen and the yi. Focus guides qi. When focusing in the lower dan tian, qi will be directed there. As qi fills the lower dan tian, it energizes the area. It energizes the organs, the glands, and all of the functions of the area. This begins the process of regeneration. When the lower dan tian is regenerated and rejuvenated, the entire body benefits.

Location

The location of where to focus our attention in the lower dan tian can vary. It is commonly described as behind the umbilicus and one to three inches below it. This is the approximate area. My suggestion is to place your attention in this area and move your attention around until you feel something. It can be a feeling of fullness, tingling, denseness, energy, or a pull. The location can change from day to day. Feeling guides the location. Indeed, feeling will be the guiding principle behind the entire practice. If you do not feel anything, continue with one of the methods, and with time and practice you will feel the qi.

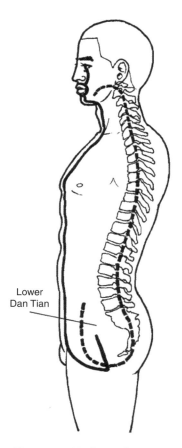

Figure 13.1 The lower dan tian

As the lower dan tian fills with qi, it is restored to a level of homeostasis or balance. As this area fills up, qi will move throughout the body according to a built-in intelligence. Nei dan is a way to enhance the flow of qi through the body. It will clear blockages, reduce excesses, supplement deficiencies, and rejuvenate the body. It can accelerate the process of rejuvenation.

BEGINNING NEI DAN

Nei dan begins with being centered and relaxed. A way to allow this feeling to occur is by focusing attention in the lower dan tian. There are a few ways to practice focusing. Two of them are now described.

Method 1: Focusing

Begin by focusing on a fixed point or area within the lower dan tian. Keep your attention on the area as you breathe naturally. Inhaling draws qi to the area. Exhaling retains the qi. This process of keeping attention on an area gathers and retains qi to the area, filling it up with qi. As the sea of qi is filled with qi, it naturally flows through the body. Practice this cultivation for one, two, three, five, eight, ten, or even 20 minutes. There is no hurry. Build up the length of your practice in a comfortable way.

Method 2: Spiraling

A second method is based on spiraling. The Taoists were cosmologists. They observed the stars and planets, and they noticed that they flowed in predictable patterns. Often we do not notice the most obvious activities around us. Earth is a planet floating in space; it is constantly spinning and in perpetual movement. Guided by the flow of the stars and planets, the ancients turned their attention inward and could feel qi moving in their body. They practiced methods to enhance internal spinning and circulation.

Spiraling causes qi to move to an area. Spiraling gathers, collects, and accumulates qi. Spiraling is a way to move qi; focusing is a way to guide qi. Combining both of these methods is a way to gather and guide qi. Begin by focusing attention in the lower dan tian. Then, after a minute or two, begin spiraling. This is done by visualizing a point that is spiraling within a small space—the size of a marble or a pearl. You can spiral clockwise or counter-clockwise. You can mix the directions up; move in one direction, and then the other direction. Keep spiraling until you feel the qi. Spiraling is commonly done for 3, 6, 9, 12, 18, 27, or 36 times. Do this in both directions, and do it until you feel qi. Be consistent in your spiraling. If you spiral nine times in one direction, then spiral nine times in the other direction.

Perform this practice until you feel qi. Select one method or combine the two: you can do only the focus method, only the spiraling method, or a combination of both methods. Practice this part of nei dan until you feel qi in the lower dan tian, which can take from a week to a few months.

THE SMALL HEAVENLY ORBIT

The small heavenly orbit is the circuit consisting of the Du and Ren channels (Figure 13.2). In this nei dan practice, guide your focus from the center of the lower dan tian down to the hui yin point (the perineum) which is about an inch above the anus. From hui yin, guide your attention/yi up to the crown, to the bai hui point (the crown center at the head vertex). This process guides attention up the Du channel. The next step is to guide your focus down the front of the body and back to the hui yin point at the perineum. In so doing, your attention has been guided down the Ren channel. Having returned to hui yin, you have completed one circuit through the small heavenly orbit.

THE SMALL HEAVENLY ORBIT

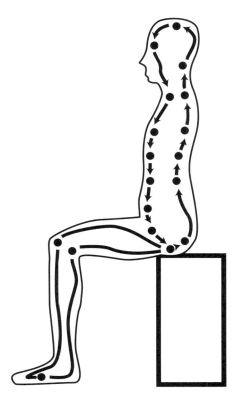

Figure 13.2 The small heavenly orbit

There are various ways to practice this nei dan. Three methods are presented below.

The first small heavenly orbit method

The first way is to connect the circulation up the Du channel and down the Ren channel with your breath:

- Throughout this nei dan, your breathing should be natural, relaxed, and gentle. Breathe from your lower dan tian.

- Begin by connecting to the center/the lower dan tian. Focus and/or spiral in the center until you feel qi.

- Inhale gently into the center. Stay relaxed, and do not change the rate of your breathing. Exhale, and gently move your attention to the hui yin area at the perineum.

- From the hui yin area, inhale up the Du channel (in front of the spine) as you count "one." Gently guide your mind up the Du channel to the crown (the bai hui point). Review the picture of the orbit to visualize the area up the back channel.

- The inhale should be completed when you arrive at the crown, at the top of the head.

- Next, guide your focus/attention down the Ren channel. Thus, during the exhale guide your attention from the crown to hui yin. Think the number "two," as you flow down the front channel.

- Yang numbers are odd and correspond to ascent. Count an odd number as you inhale up the back (the Du channel). Yin numbers are even and correspond to descent. Count an even number as you exhale down the front of the body (the Ren channel).

- Continue this circulation up the back and down the front for ten cycles. This completes one round.

- Repeat this practice for three, six, or nine rounds. Do it until you feel the qi flowing in the heavenly orbit.

A goal of the nei dan is to increase the flow of qi in the channels. Attention or focus guides qi. Moving your attention up the Du and down the Ren increases qi flow in the channels, and assists in breaking through any stagnations or blockages. This process increases energy and refines your qi. Consistent practice strengthens the internal organs, the glands, and the brain. It also refines your jing to qi, and shen. Consistent practice draws jing from the Yin area of the body up to the crown. The lower dan tian represents Yin and jing, and the upper dan tian represents Yang and shen.

Gathering Qi

Gathering qi at the end of each nei dan practice is essential for building, storing, and rejuvenating the body. There are various methods of gathering and storing, two of which are described here. Select the method that you feel is more effective. You can alternate or mix the methods.

First, when finishing the practice, gently bring your attention to the center of the lower dan tian. In the center, repeat the method used at the beginning of the practice. With your attention, spiral in clockwise and counter-clockwise directions; spiral in cycles of nine or 18 in each direction, until you feel qi gathering. The range of your spiraling can be the size of a silver dollar or a pearl. If you feel the need to expand the size, you can do it. When you finish spiraling, gently stop and keep your attention fixed in the center in the lower dan tian.

An alternative method to finish the practice is to bring your attention to the center of the lower dan tian, and then keep your attention fixed as you inhale and exhale. With your mind fixed in the center, each inhale draws qi there, and each exhale stores qi there. As you fill the center with qi, you are building the root qi of the entire body. This qi will flow into all the channels and organs to rejuvenate the body.

The second small heavenly orbit method

In this method, guide your attention/yi up the Du and down the Ren channels without connecting the circulation to your breath or counting. Circulate through the orbit at a comfortable pace. Continue the circulation through the orbit until you feel qi. Complete this meditation by gathering and collecting qi in the center of the lower dan tian.

The third small heavenly orbit method

In this method, bring your attention to major points or centers along the heavenly orbit (listed below). Begin by focusing your attention below and behind the navel. Spiral clockwise and counter-clockwise until you feel qi. The spiraling can be based on numbers (for example, multiples of nine is good) or until you feel qi. Stay balanced in the amount of clockwise and counter-clockwise spiraling. When you feel qi, gently move to the next point on the orbit and repeat the process. Continue this process for all the major points on the orbit. It may take time to open all the points. Begin by circulating through the orbit, work on some points, and then continue circulating through the orbit. Close the meditation in the normal way by gathering and storing qi in the center of the lower dan tian.

Always begin in the order listed here. You can try one or two points, then circulate through the orbit, and finally close by gathering qi in the lower dan tian. There is no rigid rule as to how many points to work on in one sitting. Be flexible.

Begin by finding the center (near the navel) in the lower dan tian. The center can range along the points and areas listed below. The range is from the navel to a few inches below and inside the body.

- *Navel*
  - Shen Que, Ren 8
  - Qi Hai, Ren 6
  - Guan Yuan, Ren 4
  - Zhong Ji, Ren 3, Perineum

  - Hui Yin, Ren 1

  - Coccyx, Chang Qiang, Du 1

  - Lumbar 2, Ming Men, Du 4

  - Thoracic Vertebra 11, Ji Zhong, Spinal Center, Adrenal Center, Du 6

  - Thoracic Vertebra 5, Shen Dao, Spirit Path, Du 11, opposite the Heart
  - Cervical Vertebra 7, Da Zhui, Big Vertebra, Du 14, opposite the throat

  - Cervical Vertebra 1, Ya Men, Gate of Muteness, Du 15

  - Crown, Bai Hui, Hundred Meetings, Du 20

  - Third eye, Yin Tang, mid-eyebrow

  - Palate, Hsuan Ying, Heavenly Pool

  - Throat, Tian Tu, Heaven's Chimney, Ren 22

- *Heart center*
  - The location is at the fourth intercostal space behind the sternum
  - Tan Zhong, Ren 17

  - Solar plexus, Zhong Wan, Middle of the Stomach, Ren 12

  - Umbilicus, Shen Que, Ren 8

After opening the point(s), circulate qi through the orbit, and then close by gathering qi in the center of the lower dan tian. Smile throughout the meditation.

Some nei dan traditions have females circulate up the Ren channel and down the Du channel. This is circulating up the front channel and down the back channel in the small heavenly orbit. I use both methods. I may start up the back and down the front, and then practice up the front and down the back channel. I finish by circulating up the back channel and down the front channel. Continue circulating in the directional flow until you feel qi. Circulating both ways can assist in balancing the Yin and Yang energies in the body. Follow how you feel. Always be guided by your feeling. Complete the meditation by gathering qi in the center of the lower dan tian.

CHAPTER 14

FIVE SHEN NEI DAN INNER MEDITATION

The Five Shen Nei Dan inner meditation is a beautiful example of applying information about the five phases into a valuable practice that can have a wonderful influence on your life. This cultivation (meditation) works on a few levels. It begins a process of turning focus/intention inward. This is a function of the yi. We develop our conscious intention and ability to turn inward, and move our life force inward and throughout the body. This ability is an essential aspect of this practice.

Balance is the key to health, vitality, and longevity. The five shen cultivation balances the energies of the body. This practice transforms life force from imbalance to balance. Table 14.1 lists the five phases correspondences used in the five shen cultivation.

PREPARATION

Begin with the inner smile meditation and then practice the small heavenly orbit for a few minutes until you feel the qi flowing in the body. When you feel the qi flowing in the small heavenly orbit, you can begin the Five Shen Nei Dan.

THE FIVE SHEN NEI DAN

Begin by sitting in a chair with your back straight and your chin tucked in gently. This posture allows the qi to flow up the back and to the brain. This is the Du channel. Turn your focus inward to the center in the lower dan tian. This is the area behind and below the navel. It is not a fixed point: wherever you feel qi, or a sensation, is where the center of the lower dan tian is located. Place your attention in the center. Allow this awareness to become stronger. Practice this meditation until you feel the qi.

Table 14.1 Five phases correspondences

Shen	Organ	Sensory organ	Sense	Temperature	Emotion	Color/Element
Shen	Heart Small Intestine	Tongue	Taste	Hot	Hastiness, impatience, hatred, arrogance	Red Fire
Zhi	Kidneys Bladder	Ears	Hearing	Cold, wet	Fear	Blue-green, black, blue Water
Hun	Liver Gallbladder	Eyes	Sight	Warm, moist	Anger, irritability, frustration	Green Wood
Po	Lungs Large Intestine	Nose	Smell	Cool, dry	Sadness, depression, loneliness	White Metal
Yi	Spleen Stomach	Mouth	Eating	Mild	Worry, pensiveness	Yellow Earth

SMILING INTO THE FIVE ORGANS

The five shen correspondences are presented in Chapter 7 of this book. Some of these correspondences are applied in this cultivation. Having a clear understanding of the physical locations of the five organs is the first step in the practice (you may need to refer to a good anatomy book).

Begin this practice by placing your attention in the Kidneys. When doing this, you are connecting your life force (qi) and the organ. The qi and the organ are integrated, and the organ is energized. This is the beginning process of creating vitality and rejuvenation. Don't just place your attention in the Kidneys—smile into the Kidneys. Smiling is an essential aspect of the practice; it creates a transformative life force that can change the emotional condition of a person.

When you feel the Kidneys filled with qi, a smiling qi, move to the next organ. Gently move your attention into the Heart. Concentrate with a relaxed body and mind, and smile into the Heart. Focus in and around the entire Heart until you feel the Heart filled with qi. When you feel the qi in the Heart, gently move to the Liver. Focus in and around the Liver until you feel the Liver full of qi. Smile into the Liver, and fill it with smiling energy. When you feel the Liver full of energy, gently move your focus into the Lungs. Smile into the Lungs. When you feel the Lungs filled with qi, gently move your attention into the Spleen. Smile into the Spleen and fill it with energy. After you have focused on the Spleen, become aware of all the five organs. Focus your attention on all the organs; feel the energy of each of the five organs. Spend up to ten minutes in this organ-awareness meditation. This meditation begins the Fusion of the Five Phases nei dan inner meditation. Finish this nei dan by gently moving your attention and qi to the lower dan tian and collect the energy.

Spend up to a few months practicing this meditation. Practice until you feel the smiling energy in all five organs. Being able to feel the qi in the organs integrates your life force and your organs (the qi and the body); it is the beginning step in self-awareness and self-realization.

THE FIVE PHASES (FIVE ELEMENTS)

This part of the nei dan includes the five elements of nature. The process is similar to the previous cultivation of smiling into the organs. Smiling into an organ connects the organ and qi. In this cultivation, we connect an organ and its element. This fusion of the body (the internal organ) and qi revitalizes the life force of the organs, and the organ itself. Continue from the smiling into the organ part of this nei dan. Begin in the Kidneys: smile into the Kidneys until you feel the qi of the Kidneys. When you feel the qi of the Kidneys, visualize and feel the energy of water. Visualize an ocean, river, lake, or a body of water you are familiar with. Feel the water. Connect your yi to the water. Bring this water awareness to your Kidneys.

Feel the water in your Kidneys. Smile into the Kidneys and feel the water qi. Continue this nei dan until you feel the water qi.

When you feel the water qi, gently move your attention to the Heart. Smile into the Heart. When you feel the smiling qi in the Heart, feel warm fire energy. A good source of fire energy is the sun. If you prefer, become aware of the nourishing heat and fire of the sun. Allow this warming fire to grow in the Heart. Smile into the fire energy in the Heart.

When you feel the fire energy of the Heart, gently move your attention to the Liver. Smile into the Liver. When you feel the smiling energy in the Liver, visualize trees in the forest or trees in some location you have experienced. Feel the trees, which is the wood element. Fill the Liver with this wood energy. Spend a few minutes or longer until you feel the wood energy.

When you feel the wood energy in the Liver, gently move your attention to the Lungs. Smile into the Lungs until you feel the smiling energy of the Lungs. The Lungs are the metal element. Visualize natural metal in our environment. Gold is a type of metal that is used in feng shui. Gold needles have been used in acupuncture. If you prefer, visualize gold. Allow this feeling of metal to manifest. Smile and guide the metal feeling into the Lungs. Fill the Lungs with metal energy. Allow this energy to grow in the Lungs. Mix the smiling energy and the metal energy in the Lungs. Sit with this metal feeling in the Lungs.

When you feel the metal energy fill the Lungs, gently move your attention to the Spleen. Smile into the Spleen. Visualize earth qi. It can be a place you have visited or lived. It can be the mountains you have experienced. Feel this mountain energy. It is ideal to practice in the natural environments that have the elements in this nei dan practice. Feel the earth energy in the Spleen. Allow this energy to fill the Spleen. Mix the earth energy and the smiling energy. Continue at this stage for a few minutes, or until you strongly feel the earth energy. Practice this nei dan for a few weeks or months, or until you feel the elements in each organ. Continue to the next part of this nei dan, or finish this nei dan by gently guiding your energy and attention to the center of the lower dan tian and collect the energy.

THE COLORS OF THE ORGANS

The five organs house the five shen. Each of the organs has a color. When the organ and its life force are balanced, the color of the organ is vibrant. In this part of the nei dan, visualize the middle center, the solar plexus area, which is the Spleen and the Stomach, filled with a yellow color. Visualize a vibrant yellow color. This is the earth phase and it is a transformer. The order in which we flow from organ to organ follows the pattern from stage one: the Kidneys, Heart, Liver, and then the Lungs.

Begin this practice by smiling into the middle center. See a glowing, yellow color in the solar plexus area. Concentrate and focus your yi in the center of the middle jiao. Settle your intention in this center until you feel a vibrant force. The middle center is the location in which all the energies of the organs will be collected and transformed. The transformed energy is a neutral qi. This qi is guided back to the organs to energize them, and begins the process of rejuvenation.

When you have completed the solar plexus (middle center) part of this nei dan, move your attention to the Kidneys. The color of the Kidneys is blue-green. Some traditions use the color black or blue. Smile into the Kidneys: visualize a vibrant blue-green color materializing there. Spend as much time as you need on this practice until you see and feel the vibrant color and qi of the Kidneys.

When you have completed the Kidneys part of this nei dan, move your attention to the Heart. The color of the Heart is red. Smile into the Heart: visualize a vibrant red color materializing there. Spend as much time as you need on this practice until you see and feel the vibrant color and qi of the Heart.

When you have completed the Heart part of this nei dan, move your attention to the Liver. The color of the Liver is green. Smile into the Liver: visualize a vibrant green color materializing there. Spend as much time as you need on this practice until you see and feel the vibrant color and qi of the Liver.

When you have completed the Liver part of this nei dan, move your attention to the Lungs. The color of the Lungs is white. Smile into the Lungs: visualize a vibrant white color materializing there. Spend as much time as you need on this practice until you see and feel the vibrant color and qi of the Lungs.

When you have completed this stage of connecting, visualizing, and feeling the vibrant energy of the organs, be aware of all the organs vibrating with their colors and qi. Spend a few minutes being with all the five organ centers.

This stage of the five shen cultivation grows the favorable energies and colors of the organs. This stage builds the life force in the organ centers, creating the strength and integrity to transform the conditioning, imprints, and emotional imbalances that may exist. We can look at this process as greeting our psycho-emotional difficulties with a smiling, loving life force. This smiling, loving energy allows for a more effective transformation.

THE FIVE PHASES SENSES

Begin this nei dan by becoming aware of your Kidneys. Focus your intention in the Kidneys. When you feel the qi of the Kidneys, move your attention (yi) to the ears. Focus on the ears: feel the life force in the ears. The ears are connected to the Kidneys. With practice you will feel the connection between the Kidneys and the ears. Spend a few minutes in this awareness of the Kidneys and the ears. This is fusion of the water correspondences, which includes the Kidneys, the ears, and the zhi spirit.

When you have completed the Kidneys part of this nei dan, move your attention to the Heart. Focus your intention in the Heart. When you feel the qi of the Heart, move your attention (yi) to the tongue. Focus on the tongue: feel the life force in the tongue. The tongue is connected to the Heart. With practice you will feel the connection between the Heart and the tongue. Spend a few minutes in this awareness of the Heart and the tongue. This is fusion of the fire correspondences, which includes the Heart, the tongue, and the shen spirit.

When you have completed the Heart part of this nei dan, move your attention to the Liver. Focus your intention in the Liver. When you feel the qi of the Liver, move your attention (yi) to the eyes. Focus on the eyes: feel the life force in the eyes. The eyes are connected to the Liver. With practice you will feel the connection between the Liver and the eyes. Spend a few minutes in this awareness of the Liver and the eyes. This is fusion of the wood correspondences, which includes the Liver, the eyes, and the hun spirit.

When you have completed the Liver part of this nei dan, move your attention to the Lungs. Focus your intention in the Lungs. When you feel the qi of the Lungs, move your attention (yi) to the nose. Focus on the nose: feel the life force in the nose. The nose is connected to the Lungs. With practice you will feel the connection between the Lungs and the nose. Spend a few minutes in this awareness of the Lungs and the nose. This is fusion of the metal correspondences, which includes the Lungs, the nose, and the po spirit.

When you have completed the Lungs part of this nei dan, move your attention to the Spleen. Focus your intention in the Spleen. When you feel the qi of the Spleen, move your attention (yi) to the mouth. Focus on the mouth: feel the life force in the mouth. The mouth is connected to the Spleen. With practice you will feel the connection between the Spleen and the mouth. Spend a few minutes in this awareness of the Spleen and the mouth. This is fusion of the earth correspondences, which includes the Spleen, the mouth, and the yi spirit. Notice that the yi is involved in each step of this nei dan. The condition of the yi is critical in our cultivation.

When you have finished this part of the nei dan, become aware of all five organs and their sensory pairings. Feel their qi. This practice is the foundation for the rest of this nei dan inner meditation.

THE FIVE PHASES TEMPERATURES

Each of the five organs is susceptible to specific temperatures. Temperature imbalances have an unfavorable influence on their own organs and their correspondences.

Begin this nei dan with smiling into the Kidneys. The temperature of the Kidneys is cold. Feel any cold in the Kidneys, or cold in the body. Allow the coldness to manifest. Spend as much time as you need until you feel the cold.

When you have completed the Kidneys part of this nei dan, move your attention to the Heart. The Heart temperature is hot. Feel the heat in the Heart, or heat in the body. Allow heat to manifest. Spend as much time as you need until you feel the heat.

When you have completed the Kidneys and Heart portion of this nei dan, simultaneously bring the cold of the Kidneys and the heat of the

Heart together. With your intention, move the cold and heat from the organs to the yellow sphere in the center of the middle jiao. This yellow sphere is the earth phase. It is the space for transforming the temperatures to a balanced, warm temperature. This transformation of temperature is the first in this fusion cultivation. Draw the temperatures, which are qi, into the middle jiao. Draw the heat from the Heart down into the top of the yellow sphere. Draw the cold from the Kidneys up into the bottom of the yellow sphere. Simultaneously spiral the energies on the outer portion of the yellow sphere, and move them to its center. When you get close to the middle of the sphere, mingle the temperatures, creating a warm temperature. Focus your attention on the center, making small circles, collecting this qi into a small, condensed qi formation. This qi formation is called a pearl, crystal, or qi ball. The process of forming this pearl will be repeated throughout this cultivation. The pearl is the refined essence of the organs and the body.

When you have completed the Kidneys and the Heart portion of this nei dan, smile into the Liver. The Liver is warm. Feel any warmth in the Liver, and warmth in the body. (It is common to feel heat in the Liver; when it is imbalanced it can heat up. If you feel heat in the Liver, continue this nei dan in the same way.) Allow the warmth to manifest. Spend as much time as you need until you feel the warmth.

When you have completed the Liver portion of this nei dan, smile into the Lungs. The Lungs are cool. Feel the coolness in the Lungs, and coolness in the body. Allow the coolness to manifest. Spend as much time as you need until you feel the coolness.

When you have completed the Liver and the Lungs portion of this nei dan, simultaneously bring the warmth of the Liver and the coolness of the Lungs together. With your intention, move the warmth and the coolness of the Liver and the Lungs to the yellow sphere in the middle jiao. This yellow sphere is the earth phase. It is the space for transforming the temperatures to a warm, balanced temperature. Guide the temperatures, which are qi, into the yellow sphere in the middle jiao. Simultaneously spiral the energies on the outer portion of the yellow sphere and move them to its center. When you get close to the middle of the sphere, mingle the temperatures, creating a nice warm temperature. Focus your attention on the center, making small circles, collecting this qi into a small, condensed pearl formation. This qi formation is also called a crystal or qi ball. This process of forming the pearl will be repeated throughout this cultivation.

Finish this part of the nei dan by feeling a mild temperature in the Spleen. Allow a mild temperature to manifest. This can be in the Spleen, as well as throughout the body. After you feel the mild temperature in the Spleen, gently guide it into the yellow sphere in the middle jiao. Mix all the temperatures in the yellow sphere. Mix them by spiraling them with your intention. Spiral 18 times one way, and 18 times the other way. You can spiral in patterns of nine. You can spiral counter-clockwise, and then clockwise. Spiral the energy (temperatures) into a small pearl shape in the center of the yellow sphere. Smile into the pearl for a few minutes.

THE EMOTIONS

In the *Su Wen* and the *Ling Shu*, the emotions and the virtues are presented. These classic texts clearly present how the body and emotions are inseparable, and that each influences the other. The Five Shen Nei Dan we are now doing is a profound practice to transform emotions. Chinese and Taoist medicine has a deep understanding of the influences of emotions. In this part of the Five Shen Nei Dan the focus is on emotions.

Part 1: The Kidneys

Begin this nei dan by becoming aware of your Kidneys. Focus your intention in the Kidneys. When you feel the qi of the Kidneys, allow any fear to manifest. Allow any repressed, suppressed, or existing fear to become conscious. Focus on this fear. Emotions are energy, and in this practice we seek to transform this energy to its original nature. When you feel the fear, move it into the blue-green sphere at the lower portion of the lower dan tian. This area is at Ren 1, hui yin, the Meeting of Yin. Figure 14.1 shows the collection points area. It is at the perineum. In five phases theory and Chinese medicine, fire is Yang and water is Yin. They are Shao Yin pairs. It is the fire correspondences that will assist in transforming the fear. The next part of this cultivation occurs in the Heart.

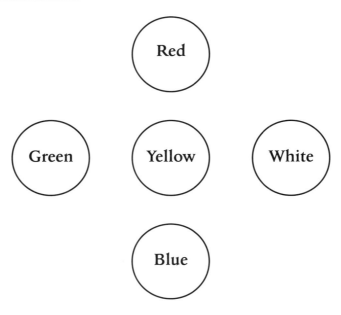

Figure 14.1 The collection points

Part 2: The Heart

When you have completed the Kidneys part of this nei dan, gently move your attention to the Heart. When you feel the Heart qi, allow any hastiness, arrogance, impatience, and hatred to manifest. When we bury our emotions deep inside our body and mind, they influence deep parts of our being. In Chinese medical terminology, they influence the yuan level. This is the jing (essence) level and it is our constitution. To change the essence level, we need to allow this energy (emotion) to come to the surface, to be transformed to a neutral qi. When you feel these emotions, move them into the red sphere in the Heart center area (the location is at Ren 17, tan zhong).

Part 3: Fusion of the Kidneys and the Heart

When you have completed the Kidneys/zhi and Heart/shen portion of this nei dan, simultaneously bring the emotional energy of the Kidneys and the Heart together. With your intention, move the fear and the hastiness, arrogance, impatience, and hatred together into the yellow sphere in the middle center. The process is similar to that used in the temperature part of this nei dan. Guide the emotional energy of the Heart down into the top of the yellow sphere. And then guide the emotional energy of the Kidneys up to the bottom of the yellow sphere. Simultaneously spiral these emotional energies on the outer portion of the yellow sphere, moving to its center. The movement is from the outer to the inner. As you spiral the emotional energies towards the center, their energies begin to mingle. When you get close to the middle of the sphere, focus on combining these energies together. This yellow sphere of the transforming earth phase allows the emotional energy to transform to its natural, balanced life force. Finish this part of the nei dan by collecting this qi into a small, condensed pearl formation. Smile to this pearl for a few minutes.

Part 4: The Liver

The next part of this cultivation is to harmonize the Liver/hun and the Lungs/po. Begin this nei dan by bringing your attention to the Liver. When you feel the Liver qi, allow any anger, irritability, and frustration to manifest. Be aware of these emotions. When you feel this emotional energy in the Liver, gently guide it into the green sphere at the Liver collection area. This area is below the Liver at the right side of the body. The area is on the nipple line, at the level of the navel. Draw a line from the navel laterally to a line flowing down from the nipple line. The intersection of these two lines is where the green sphere is located. The area is at the acupuncture point, Spleen 15, Daheng, Great Horizontal. Spiral the emotional energy in the green sphere to collect it there.

Part 5: The Lungs

The next step in this cultivation is to cultivate the Lungs. Begin this nei dan by bringing your attention to the Lungs. When you feel the Lung qi, allow any sadness, depression, grief, and loneliness to manifest. Be aware of these emotions. When you feel this emotional energy of the Lungs, gently guide it into the white sphere at the Lung collection area. This collection area is at the left side of the body, on the nipple line, at the level of the navel. Draw a line from the navel laterally to a line flowing down from the nipple line. The intersection of these two lines is where the white sphere is located.

The area is at the acupuncture point, Spleen 15, Daheng, Great Horizontal. Spiral the emotional energy in the white sphere to collect it there.

Part 6: Fusion of the Liver and the Lungs

When you have completed the Liver and Lungs portion of this nei dan, simultaneously bring the emotional energy of the Liver and the Lungs together. With your intention, move the emotional energy of the Liver and Lungs into the yellow sphere in the middle jiao. The process is similar to that used with the Kidneys and the Heart. Guide the emotional energy of the Liver and the Lungs into the yellow sphere in the middle jiao. Simultaneously spiral these emotional energies at the outer portion of the yellow sphere, moving to its center. The movement is from the outer to the inner. As you spiral the emotional energies towards the center, their energies begin to mingle. When you get close to the middle of the sphere, focus on combining these energies together. This yellow sphere of the transforming earth phase allows the emotional energy to transform to its natural, balanced, life force. The transformed emotional energy of the Kidneys and the Heart are in the yellow sphere; the transformed energy of the Liver and the Lungs is now mixed with these energies. There is a synergy occurring as more of the energies are mixed together. Finish this part of the nei dan by collecting this qi into a small, condensed pearl formation. Smile to this pearl for a few minutes.

Part 7: The Spleen

Working with the Spleen is the last step of this part of the nei dan practice. Begin this cultivation by becoming aware of your Spleen. Focus your intention in the Spleen. When you feel the qi of the Spleen, allow any worry, excessive pensiveness, and obsessiveness to manifest. Focus on these emotions and imbalances of the Spleen (yi). When you feel these imbalances, move them to the yellow sphere in the middle center. Spiral this energy from the outer aspect of the yellow sphere towards the center. Using your yi, spiral in the yellow sphere. When you continually spiral in the yellow sphere, all the energies of the Kidneys, Heart, Liver, Lungs, and Spleen are fused together into one energy: this is the pearl.

There is a synergy that is created in this nei dan. This process transforms the individual organ and the elemental energy into a refined life force, which rejuvenates the body. This is inner medicine. The next stage of this cultivation is a powerful rejuvenation nei dan. It is a powerful self-healing practice.

REJUVENATING THE ORGANS AND THE FIVE SHEN

The refined essences of the organs are now in the form of a pearl. This energy is a purified life force, and can rejuvenate our body and mind. This final part of the nei dan is to return this refined life force to the internal organs to vitalize and rejuvenate them. This rejuvenation nei dan follows the creation cycle of the five phases. The flow from organ to organ is also called the creation/nourishing five phases cycle. This nei dan practice is guiding the energy or life force (the pearl) from organ to organ, until all the organs are nourished. The order is the Kidneys, Liver, Heart, Spleen, and Lungs. This pattern is repeated multiple times until you feel the life force in each organ.

Begin this nei dan by smiling and bringing your attention and the pearl into the Kidneys. Allow the pearl to expand to cover all of the Kidneys. Gently move your attention throughout the Kidneys, filling the Kidneys with a blue-green color. Smile into the Kidneys for a few minutes, until you feel the Kidney qi. When you decide to continue to the next part of this nei dan, gather the Kidney energy into a pearl and move it to the Liver.

The Liver is a green color. When you move the blue-green pearl of the Kidneys into the Liver, smile into the Liver and allow the blue-green pearl to transform into a green-colored pearl. Allow this green pearl to expand to cover the entire Liver. Smile into the Liver and feel this vibrant Liver qi. When you decide to continue to the next part of this nei dan, gather the Liver energy into a pearl and move it to the Heart.

The Heart is a red color. When you move the green pearl of the Liver into the Heart, smile into the Heart and allow the green pearl to transform into a red-colored pearl. Allow this red pearl to expand to cover the entire Heart. Smile into the Heart and feel this vibrant Heart qi. When you decide to continue to the next part of this nei dan, gather the Heart energy into a pearl and move it to the Spleen.

The Spleen is a yellow color. When you move the red pearl of the Heart into the Spleen, smile into the Spleen and allow the red pearl to transform into a yellow-colored pearl. Allow this yellow pearl to expand to cover the entire Spleen. Smile into the Spleen and feel this vibrant Spleen qi. When you decide to continue to the next part of this nei dan, gather the Spleen energy into a pearl and move it to the Lungs.

The Lungs are a white color. When you move the yellow pearl of the Spleen into the Lungs, smile into the Lungs and allow the yellow pearl to transform into a white-colored pearl. Allow this white pearl to expand to cover the entire Lungs. Smile into the Lungs and feel this vibrant Lung qi. You can end this nei dan by moving the pearl to the lower dan tian, and spiral it there to collect the qi. If you prefer to continue the nei dan, repeat the cycle three or more times. It is common practice to repeat in multiples of three. Always finish the nei dan by collecting the energy in the lower dan tian.

A powerful way to end this nei dan is to circulate the qi/pearl in the small heavenly orbit three, six, or nine times. This orbit circulation brings a refined and potent life force into the Ren and Du channels. It benefits the entire body. If you have read and practiced the eight extraordinary channels nei dan presented in my book, *Eight Extraordinary Channels—Qi Jing Ba Mai: A Handbook for Clinical Practice and Nei Dan Inner Meditation*, move the pearl through all the eight extraordinary channels in the pattern presented in the book.

The Fusion of the Five Phases nei dan is a profound inner meditation that clears, transforms, and refines our life force. We have three treasures: the physical, mental, and spiritual aspects of our life. From a Chinese medical perspective, the three treasures are jing, qi, and shen. This five shen cultivation has a profound influence on the imbalances that occur in our life, and within each of the three treasures. Imbalances can exist within temperatures, tastes, sensory organs, and emotions. This Five Shen Nei Dan can transform the effects of the rough, and its imprints on our life.

Becoming *aware* is a major aspect of the transformation process. This nei dan focuses on creating awareness on each of the correspondences that are in this practice. Becoming aware allows the imbalance to become conscious, and provides the opportunity to understand (from an experiencing perspective) and transform the energies. Part of this process is to restore the life force to its normal, natural condition. This is called the yuan (original) condition. Instead of trying to remove the imbalanced energy from the body, we seek to transform the life force. In this way we do not reduce our life force, but retain it and use it to rejuvenate the body.

The Chinese perceived that each person consisted of physical, emotional, and spiritual energies. And each person has a level of freedom to decide where to place their attention and their life force. Where we focus our life force manifests the type of life we experience. We have the free will to focus our attention and create a mindfulness of how we want to live life. The *process of focus* is the beginning of transformation and nei dan.

The Five Shen Nei Dan presented here has a profound influence on emotions. In transforming emotions, we become more aware of our energy. When imbalances in our emotional life absorb our life force, we have less energy to focus on our spiritual life. A benefit of this nei dan is that it assists in releasing us from attachments to our emotions and allows us to focus or become aware of our spiritual nature. The spirit is always with us. A goal of nei dan is to clear the rough (stresses, emotions, imprints, and conditioning) in our life that requires our life force to maintain them. When this rough is cleared, we can naturally become aware of our spirit. This awareness will become natural with cultivation. In a way a new conditioning occurs: it is living from spirit. The duration required to clear the rough differs with each person. From my experience as a practitioner and teacher, with practice this Five Shen Nei Dan is a potent way to clear the rough, allowing the natural awareness of spirit, and the Tao within.

CONCLUSION

The early practitioners of acupuncture were medical physicians. They treated a wide range of health conditions, creating a comprehensive system of natural healing which included five major channel systems. It was their experience that each channel system more effectively treated the conditions in their locations than one channel system treating all the areas of the body. The divergent channels (separate channels) are presented in Chapter 11 of the *Ling Shu*. Only the pathways are presented. Most interestingly, the *Ling Shu* practitioners suggest that the superior physician knows they are difficult to understand, but are essential to learn. The text also suggests that an extraordinary number of diseases can manifest in these channels. A goal of this book is to work out theories that contribute towards understanding these channels, and learn how to apply them in clinical practice. I have found that these channels have substantially increased my clinical effectiveness. I hope you will include these channels in your practice. If you have questions or feedback about this book please contact me through my website: www.healingqi.com.

ENDNOTES

1. Ni, M. (1995) *The Yellow Emperor's Classic of Medicine: A New Translation of the Neijing Suwen with Commentary*, Chapter 27. Boston, MA: Shambhala.
2. Wu, J. (2002) *Ling Shu or The Spiritual Pivot*, Chapter 71. Hawaii: University of Hawaii Press.
3. Ni, M. (1995) *The Yellow Emperor's Classic of Medicine: A New Translation of the Neijing Suwen with Commentary*, Chapter 50. Boston, MA: Shambhala.
4. Wu, J. (2002) *Ling Shu or The Spiritual Pivot*, Chapter 3. Hawaii: University of Hawaii Press.
5. Wu, J. (2002) *Ling Shu or The Spiritual Pivot*, Chapter 5. Hawaii: University of Hawaii Press.
6. Wu, J. (2002) *Ling Shu or The Spiritual Pivot*, Chapter 11. Hawaii: University of Hawaii Press.
7. Wu, J. (2002) *Ling Shu or The Spiritual Pivot*, Chapter 11. Hawaii: University of Hawaii Press.
8. Wu, J. (2002) *Ling Shu or The Spiritual Pivot*, Chapter 5. Hawaii: University of Hawaii Press.
9. Wu, J. (2002) *Ling Shu or The Spiritual Pivot*, Chapter 5. Hawaii: University of Hawaii Press.
10. Wu, J. (2002) *Ling Shu or The Spiritual Pivot*, Chapter 10. Hawaii: University of Hawaii Press.
11. Discussed in Wang, Z., and Wang, J. (2007) *Ling Shu Acupuncture*, Irvine, CA: Ling Shu Press.
12. Wu, J. (2002) *Ling Shu or The Spiritual Pivot*, Chapter 1. Hawaii: University of Hawaii Press.
13. Ni, M. (1995) *The Yellow Emperor's Classic of Medicine: A New Translation of the Neijing Suwen with Commentary*, Chapter 5. Boston, MA: Shambhala.

14. Ni, M. (1995) *The Yellow Emperor's Classic of Medicine: A New Translation of the Neijing Suwen with Commentary*, Chapter 5. Boston, MA: Shambhala.

15. Wu, J. (2002) *Ling Shu or The Spiritual Pivot*, Chapter 8. Hawaii: University of Hawaii Press.

16. Ni, H.C. (1995) "The Shrine of the Eternal Breath of Tao." *The Complete Works of Lao Tzu*, Chapter 11. Santa Monica, CA: Sevenstar Communications.

17. Ni, M. (1995) *The Yellow Emperor's Classic of Medicine: A New Translation of the Neijing Suwen with Commentary*, Chapter 63. Boston, MA: Shambhala.

18. Ni, M. (1995) *The Yellow Emperor's Classic of Medicine: A New Translation of the Neijing Suwen with Commentary*, Chapter 50. Boston, MA: Shambhala.

19. Wu, J. (2002) *Ling Shu or The Spiritual Pivot*, Chapter 3. Hawaii: University of Hawaii Press.

20. Wu, J. (2002) *Ling Shu or The Spiritual Pivot*, Chapter 5. Hawaii: University of Hawaii Press.

21. Wu, J. (2002) *Ling Shu or The Spiritual Pivot*, Chapter 7. Hawaii: University of Hawaii Press.

22. Wu, J. (2002) *Ling Shu or The Spiritual Pivot*, Chapter 1. Hawaii: University of Hawaii Press.

BIBLIOGRAPHY

Johnson, J.A. (2000) *Chinese Medical Qi Gong Therapy.* Pacific Grove, CA: International Institute of Medical Qi Gong.

Lu, H. (1985) *A Complete Translation of The Yellow Emperor's Classic of Internal Medicine and the Difficult Classic.* Vancouver: Academy of Oriental Heritage.

Luk, C., and Yu, K.Y. (1999) *Taoist Yoga: Alchemy and Immortality.* San Francisco, CA: Red Wheel/Weiser.

Maciocia, G. (2006) *The Channels of Acupuncture: Clinical Use of the Secondary Channels and the Eight Extraordinary Vessels.* Oxford: Churchill Livingstone.

Ni, M. (1995) *The Yellow Emperor's Classic of Medicine: A New Translation of Neijing Suwen with Commentary.* Boston, MA: Shambhala.

Ni, Y. (1996) *Navigating the Channels of Traditional Chinese Medicine.* San Diego, CA: Complementary Medicine Press.

Shima, M., and Chace, C. (2001) *The Channel Divergences: Deeper Pathways of the Web.* Boulder, CO: Blue Poppy Press.

Twicken, D. (2002) *Treasures of Tao.* Bloomington, IN: iUniverse.

Twicken, D. (2011) *I Ching Acupuncture—The Balance Method: Clinical Applications of the Ba Gua and I Ching.* London: Singing Dragon.

Twicken, D. (2013) *Eight Extraordinary Channels—Qi Jing Ba Mai: A Handbook for Clinical Practice and Nei Dan Inner Meditation.* London: Singing Dragon.

Van Nghi, T., Dzung, T., and Nguyen, C. (2005–2010) *Huang Di Nei Jing, Ling Shu* (three volumes). Sugar Grove, NC: Jung Tao School of Classic Chinese Medicine.

Veith, I. (1966) *The Yellow Emperor's Classic of Internal Medicine.* Berkeley, CA: University of California Press.

Wang, Z., and Wang, J. (2007) *Ling Shu Acupuncture.* Irvine, CA: Ling Shu Press.

Wu, J. (2002) *Ling Shu or The Spiritual Pivot.* Hawaii: University of Hawaii Press.

Wu, N., and Wu, A. (2002) *Yellow Emperor's Canon of Internal Medicine.* Beijing: China Science Technology Press.

Yang, C. (2004) *A Systematic Classic of Acupuncture and Moxibustion.* Boulder, CO: Blue Poppy Press.

INDEX

Abyss of the Armpit 36, 38, 40
acupuncture channel system
    channel types 17–18
    circulation of vital substances 180
    divergent channels as integral part of 21
    influences of time and space 20
    as pathway for circulation 180
    pathways 27
    qualities and relationships within 44–5
    relationship with human body 103, 131
acupuncture practice 131–3, 152
alchemy
    defining 181
    internal 120–1, 173
    nei dan as 183
anatomical structures
    and divergent channels 147–8
    link with vital substances 110
    paired 50
anger case study 163–4
animal spirit 115, 174
Arm Bright Channel 40
Arm Bright Yang 40
Arm Major Yang 36
Arm Major Yin 40
Arm Minor Yang 38
Arm Minor Yin 36
Arm Pericardium 38
astrology *see* Chinese medical astrology
awareness 118, 120, 121, 129, 210–11

Ba Gua *see* Early Heaven Ba Gua
back pain case study 161–2
back pain treatment 159
balance
    Ba Gua 56
    of controlling cycle 116, 126
    five shen cultivation 197
    importance in Chinese medicine 121, 175
    internal 174
    shen and po 126–7
    trigrams 54–5
beginnings *see* roots and ends
birth hours 111
Bladder
    connecting channel conditions 98
    divergent channel
        conditions 83
        distribution 63–4
        ends and beginnings 146
        pathways 28, 29–30, 158
        points 68, 71–2, 77, 83, 150, 170
        roots and ends 85, 147
        sequence 40, 42, 51, 69
        treatment assistance 158, 159, 160, 161–2
        as Yang 64
    major channel conditions 92
    muscle channel
        conditions 106
        cycle 105
        month 104
    organ
        conditions 96
        five shen and correspondences 130, 198
        hour of birth 111
        lower dan tian 178
        nourishing qi 102
        resonances 115
        wei qi 105
        as Yang 59

blame case study 166–8
blood
    channel controlling 91
    circulation 151, 159
    emotions stored in 97, 124, 179
    needle for 135, 138
    and Spleen 123–4, 130, 179
    storehouse of 115
    as vital substance 27
    as Yin 174
blood channels *see* connecting channels
bloodletting 73, 77, 156, 160, 163
bones
    connections 45, 109, 148
    controlling channel 93
    nature of 109–10, 150–1
    and needling 21, 132
    as Yin 148
Broken Dish 38, 40, 93, 102, 106–7

centers of the body 177, 184, 193–5
chaos 120, 128, 147
chest
    as area of ending 85, 146, 147
    conditions 90, 93, 94–5, 96, 97, 98, 107
    divergent channel points 79, 81, 83, 84
    and Heart shen 119
    shu points of 119
China's four great traditions 175
Chinese dynasties 15–16
Chinese medical astrology 110–11
Chinese medicine
    applied to philosophy 13
    assisting change 118

217

Chinese medicine *cont.*
  on balance 121
  on bones 109, 110
  circulation of water and vital substances 180
  early practitioner beliefs 17, 23, 67
  essence of 14, 23, 156, 161
  essential aspect of 19–20, 44–5, 101
  first energy in body 183
  priority given to organs 94
  relationship between earth and water 128–9
  understanding of psychological and spiritual aspects 176
chronic fatigue
  case study 164–5
  treatment 160
Classic of Acupuncture and Moxibustion 17, 22
clearing stasis *see* dredging
clinical acupuncture framework 155–6
conditions
  according to hour of birth 111
  appropriate channel for treating 131–2
  of connecting channels 98, 160
  divergent channels
    ability to treat 44–5, 99, 109–10, 155
    and main points 83–4
    treating the pathways 158
  of internal organs 70, 94–7
  main ways to view 89–90
  of major channels 90–4, 149
  of muscle channels 106–9, 150
  needles for treating 134–6, 138, 142–3, 148–9
  shen and Yin organs 176
confluences *see* junctions
confluent points 68, 71, 73, 75, 77, 79, 81, 83–4, 85, 110, 150, 157, 170
connecting channels
  in anger treatment 156, 163
  and divergent channels 43–4, 99
  needle for treating 135, 138
  as part of acupuncture system 18
  pathology 97–9
  at superficial/wei layer 132
  supporting 160
  as treatment 122

connecting points 73, 77, 156, 160, 163, 166, 169
contra-lateral needling 143
correspondences
  and awareness 210–11
  between conditions 108
  on Early Heaven Ba Gua 63
  familiarity with 125
  five phases 23, 198
  five shen 114–15, 130, 176
  fusion of 202–3
  Heaven and Earth trigrams 57
  I Ching 52
  nine needles 142
  organ 70, 174–5, 183
  pairings 50
  po 122
  as presented in Ling Shu 18–19
  as relationships 19–20
  three forces 52
  yi 123
cosmic map 17
cycles
  Chinese medical astrology 110–11
  controlling 116–17, 126
  daily clock 101–3, 146, 147
  fifty 147
  five phases creation 49, 58–9, 125–6, 209
  muscle channels 104–6
  nourishing qi 101–3, 147
  of time 20, 101–11
  wei qi 105–6

dan tian *see* three dan tian
deep layer 44, 69–70, 102–3, 109–10, 132–3, 142, 143, 149, 150
depression case study 168–9
depths of acupuncture 143, 149
diamond in the rough 174, 176, 177
diseases
  channels as location of 21, 89, 213
  in divergent channels 21, 43
  transference 43–4
  see also conditions
distal needling 148–9
divergent channels
  advice about 22, 27
  and anatomical structures 147–8
  clearing pathogenic factors 103, 150–1

  clinical applications of 103, 155–60
  connection to layers 43–4, 109–10, 132, 142, 143, 149
  constituents 67–8
  diseases in 21, 43
  and emotions 149
  as energy fields 155
  flexibility 23
  function 21
  fundamental qualities 68–70
  and muscle channels 105–6
  needles for 138
  pathways 27–40, 158
  points 71–82
    and channel conditions 83–4
    confluent 110, 170
    pathway 170
    and river patterns 149–50
    roots and ends 85
    sequence 40–2
    sequencing theories *see* Early Heaven Ba Gua; He Tu
  treatment
    of all channels 13, 21–2, 44–5, 99, 110, 133, 158–60
    case studies 161–9
    framework 156–8
    supporting spiritual realization 129
Dou Han Qing 99
dredging 69, 90, 141, 151, 158
Du channel 28, 98, 102, 160, 187, 190, 191–2, 195, 197, 210

Early Heaven Ba Gua
  explanation of 52–5
  and opposite channel pairs 63–5
  structure 56–7
  and Yin-Yang acupuncture channel pairs 57–62
ears
  as area of ending 85, 146, 147
  conditions 93, 108
  and Pericardium divergent channel 38
  relation to Kidney 121, 198, 202
Earth
  as below the waist in body 150
  as center of He Tu 49–51

confluent points 71, 73, 75, 77, 79, 81
controlled by Wood 116, 125
controller of Water 116, 129
as Foot Yang channel 42
lower dan tian 179
on meridian clock 102
and nourishing qi cycle 103
as one of five phases 113
opposite channel pairs 63
pattern of channel placement 59–62
position in Ba Gua 54–7
reinforcing Metal 144, 147
relation to yellow 198, 204, 207, 208
relation to yi 125, 130, 198, 203
relation to zhi 128
relationship with Heaven and humanity 18–19, 52, 179
Stomach and Spleen 51, 123, 125, 128–9, 130, 179, 184, 198, 200, 201, 203
and Taoist philosophy 180
at third junction 41, 68
trigram 54, 64
as Yang 59
as Yin 58
emotions
    case study 168–9
    connecting channels for treating 97, 160
    and divergent channels 149, 156
    five shen 116–17, 176–7, 198
    nei dan 174–5, 184, 205–9, 211
    inseparable relationship with body 113
    needle influencing 138
    and po 122, 130
    seven 20
    Stomach and Spleen 123, 130
    transference of 125
    unresolved 102–3
    and yi 124, 130, 179
ends *see* roots and ends
entering and exiting principle 145
exogenous factors 20
extraordinary channels 44, 45, 102–3, 109, 125, 132, 148, 160, 210
eyes
    as area of ending 85, 146, 147

conditions 90, 92, 93, 96, 106, 107, 108, 122
correspondences 198
Gallbladder divergent channel 32
Heart divergent channel 36, 77, 84
Liver opens to 122, 202
Spleen divergent channel 75, 84
Stomach divergent channel 34

fangshi (*fang-shih*) 173
fifth junction 37, 38, 41, 84
fifty cycles 147
Fire
    controlled by Water 116, 129
    controller of Metal 116
    directional number 50, 51
    at fifth junction 41
    at fourth junction 41
    as Hand Yin channels 42
    Heart 51, 126, 130, 165–6, 198, 200, 202
    Liver 22
    on meridian clock 102
    as one of five phases 113
    opposite channel pairs 63
    pattern of channel placement 59–62
    Pericardium 51, 79
    position in Ba Gua 54–6
    relation to red 198
    relation to shen 130, 198, 202
    San Jiao 51
    Small Intestine 51, 59, 130, 198
    Stomach 152, 159
    as top of He Tu 49, 51
    trigram 54, 64
    volatile and explosive nature of 119
    as Yang 59, 205
    as Yin 58
first junction 29, 30, 40, 83
five phases
    correspondences 23, 198
    cycles 125–6
    creation 49, 58–9, 209
    five elements of nature 113–14, 199–200
    fusion of 183, 184, 199, 210
    within He Tu 49, 51
    as major aspect of nei dan 173
    senses 202–3
    temperatures 203–5

five shen 117–25
    correspondences 114–15, 130
    and emotions 116–17, 176–7
    group dynamics 125–9
    housed in Yin organs 169
    imbalances 125
    inherent qualities 116
    as insight 176–7
    and rejuvenation of organs 209–10
    relation to organs 114
    resonances 114–15
    storehouses 115
    unfolding of, in body 113–14
Five Shen Nei Dan 22–3
    colors of organs 201–2
    emotions 174, 205–9, 211
    five phases 199–200
        correspondences 198
        senses 202–3
        temperatures 203–4
    five shen and organ rejuvenation 209–10
    practice 197–8
    preparation 197
    smiling into the five organs 198–9
    transformation 180–1, 210–11
focus 128–9, 187–8, 189, 211
Foot Jue Yin 41, 42, 94, 107
Foot Minor Yin 107
Foot Shao Yang 41, 42, 93–4, 106
Foot Shao Yin 40, 42, 92–3
Foot Tai Yang 40, 42, 92, 106, 162
Foot Tai Yin 41, 91, 107
Foot Yang channels 42
Foot Yang Ming 41, 91, 106–7
Foot Yin channels 42
forces, three 52
fourth junction 35, 36, 41, 84
"from beginning to end" principle 50, 57, 143, 145
Fu Xi 47
Fusion of the Five Phases 183, 184, 199, 210–11
    see also Five Shen Nei Dan

Gallbladder
    connecting channel conditions 98
    divergent channel
        conditions 83
        distribution 63–4
        ends and beginnings 146

Gallbladder *cont.*
  pathways 31–2
  points 73–4, 77, 79, 83, 170
  roots and ends 85, 147
  sequence 41, 42, 51
  treatment assistance 156, 160, 163–4, 166, 169
  as Yang 64
  major channel conditions 93–4
  muscle channel
    conditions 106
    cycle 105
    month 104
  organ
    conditions 96
    five shen and correspondences 130, 198
    hour of birth 111
    nourishing qi 102
    resonances 115
    wei qi 105
    as Yang 59
Great luo of Spleen connecting channel 98
grief case study 168–9
gua sha 73, 135, 156, 159, 166
guest and host treatment 50, 99

Han dynasty 52, 117, 151
hand divergent channels 42
Hand Jue Yin 41, 42, 93, 109
Hand Shao Yang 41, 42, 93, 108
Hand Shao Yin 41, 42, 92, 109
Hand Tai Yang 41, 42, 92, 108
Hand Tai Yin 41, 42, 90, 108
Hand Yang Ming 41, 42, 90, 108
harmony 174
He Tu 47–51, 65
head
  as area of ending 85, 147
  conditions 92, 96, 98, 143
  crown 190, 192
  upper dan tian 179
Heart
  connecting channel conditions 98
  divergent channel
    conditions 84
    distribution 63–4
    pathways 35–6
    points 77–8, 84, 170
    sequence 41, 42, 51
    treatment assistance 165–6

  as Yin 64
  emotions 116, 206–7
  major channel conditions 92
  muscle channel
    conditions 109
    cycle 105
    month 104
  in nei dan meditation 174, 199, 200, 201, 202, 203–4, 206–7, 209
  organ
    center 184, 185, 195
    conditions 90, 91, 92–3, 95
    correspondences 130, 198
    emotions 206
    hour of birth 111
    middle dan tian 179
    nourishing qi 102
    qi 183
    resonances 114
    as shen 116, 118–19, 126–7, 129, 130, 176–7, 198
    as storehouse 115
    upper dan tian 181
    wei qi 105
    as Yin 58, 113
Heaven
  above the waist 150
  in Early Heaven Ba Gua 56–7, 63
  location of confluent points 71, 73, 75, 77, 79, 81
  on needling 151
  nourishing qi cycle 103
  relation to humanity and Earth 52, 67
  relationship with humanity and Earth 18–19, 52, 179
  upper dan tian 179
  Yang trigram 54–5, 57, 64
  see also small heavenly orbit
hexagrams 52–3
hour of birth 111
Hua Tuo 151
human soul 115, 174
humanity
  and cosmos 114
  and Heaven and Earth 18–19, 52, 179
  and nature 17–18, 20, 113, 173
  and universe 67, 173
hun 121–2
  controlled by po 116
  controller of yi 116
  correspondences 130, 198
  group dynamics 126–8

  harmonizing 207
  imbalances 73, 114, 121, 122, 160
  inherent qualities 116, 177
  Liver as shelter of 115
  treating repressed 163–4
  see also Liver

I Ching 52
imaging 52, 57
imbalances
  channel flow 43–4, 94, 97
  chaos reflecting 147
  and dan tian 177, 179
  of emotions 177, 187, 202, 208, 211
  expression 118
  Liver and Gallbladder 163
  and nourishing qi cycle 103
  post-natal to deep yuan 103
  shen 119–22, 125–6, 210
  of Spleen 208
  temperature 203
inner map of the human body 17–20, 27
inner smile meditation 184–6, 197
insights 175–7
insomnia case study 165–6
internal organs
  conditions of 94–7
  correspondences 198
  five yin 113
  influence of divergent channels 44, 70, 85
  needles for treating 138
  rejuvenation 209–11
  supporting 159

jing
  in bones 109, 150
  earth shaping form of 129
  as essence 180, 206
  Kidneys storing 178
  lower dan tian 192
  needles and channels 138
  as one of three treasures 22, 67
  as qi in dense form 181
  seeking shen 129, 181
  treatable by divergent channels 45
  as vital substance 27
  and zhi shen 119, 120
Jue Yin 85, 105, 146, 147
junctions 29, 31, 33, 35, 37, 39, 40–2, 68, 70, 83–4

Kidney
  center 184
  connecting channel conditions 98
  divergent channel
    conditions 83
    distribution 63–4
    ends and beginnings 146
    pathways 28, 29–30, 161
    points 68, 71–2, 83, 150, 152, 170
    roots and ends 85, 147
    sequence 40, 42, 51, 69
    treatment assistance 158, 159, 160, 161, 162
    as Yin 64
  emotions 116, 205–7
  fusion with Heart 206–7
  major channel conditions 92–3
  muscle channel
    conditions 107
    cycle 105
    month 104
  in nei dan meditation 180, 185, 198–204, 209
  organ
    conditions 96, 114
    correspondences 130, 198
    hour of birth 111
    lower dan tian 178, 180, 181, 187
    nourishing qi 102
    qi 183
    resonances 115
    as storehouse 115
    wei qi 105
    as Yang 178
    as Yin 59, 113, 178
    as zhi 116, 119–21, 128–9, 130, 167, 176–7, 198
knees
  conditions 91, 92, 94, 106, 107
  originating point 69
  treating at crease 143

Lake 54, 55, 56, 63, 64
lancet 157, 160
Large Intestine
  connecting channel
    conditions 98
    treatment assistance 168–9
  divergent channel
    conditions 84
    distribution 63–4
    pathways 39–40
    points 75, 81–2, 84, 170
    sequence 41, 42, 51
    treatment assistance 50, 169
    as Yang 64
  major channel
    conditions 90
    and po 122
    treatment assistance 168–9
  muscle channel
    conditions 108
    cycle 105
    month 104
  organ
    conditions 95
    five shen and correspondences 130, 198
    hour of birth 111
    nourishing qi 102
    resonances 115
    wei qi 105
    as Yang 59
Later Heaven Ba Gua 47
layers of the body see three layers of the body
Leg Bright Yang 34
Leg Major Yang 30
Leg Major Yin 34
Leg Minor Yang 32
Leg Minor Yin 30
Leg Shrinking Yin 32
Ling Shu 17, 22, 27, 44–5, 173–4
Liver
  connecting channel conditions 98
  divergent channel
    conditions 83
    distribution 63–4
    ends and beginnings 146
    pathways 31–2
    points 73–4, 83, 170
    roots and ends 85, 147
    sequence 41, 42, 51
    treatment assistance 22, 156, 160, 163–4
    as Yin 64
  emotions 116, 117, 207, 208
  fusion with Lungs 208
  major channel conditions 94
  muscle channel
    conditions 107
    cycle 105
    month 104
  in nei dan meditation 174, 185, 199, 200, 201, 202–3, 204, 207–8, 209
  organ
    conditions 97
    correspondences 130, 198
    hour of birth 111
    as hun 114, 116, 121–2, 176, 177, 198
    nourishing qi 102
    qi 183, 207, 209
    resonances 114
    as storehouse 115
    wei qi 105
    as Yin 58
  lower dan tian 178, 179–80, 181, 187–9
Lung
  connecting channel conditions 98
  divergent channel
    distribution 63–4
    pathways 39–40
    points 81–2, 84, 170
    sequence 41, 42, 51
    treatment assistance 50, 169
    as Yin 64
  emotions 116, 117, 207–8
  fusion with Liver 208
  major channel conditions 90
  muscle channel
    conditions 108
    cycle 105
    month 104
  in nei dan meditation 174, 185, 199, 200, 201, 203, 204, 207–8, 210
  organ
    center 184
    conditions 94–5
    correspondences 130, 198
    hour of birth 111
    middle dan tian 179
    needles for treating 134, 138
    nourishing qi 102
    as po 116, 122–3, 126, 130, 168, 176, 177, 198
    qi 183
    resonances 114
    as storehouse 115
    treatment assistance 144, 147, 165
    upper dan tian 181
    wei qi 105
    as Yin 58, 114, 169
luo channels see connecting channels
luo points see connecting points
Luo Shu 17, 47

major channels 89–90, 144
  analogy with Earth's rivers 19
  anger influencing 125
  categorization 58–9
  conditions 90–4
  as extension of organs 149
  imbalances in 103
  middle level 143, 144
  needle for 135, 138
  relationship with divergent channels 44, 69–70, 85
  supporting 159, 165
  treatment assistance 168
  Yin-Yang pairs 145
  ying layer 132, 142, 149
Mantak Chia 174
masters of the method/formula 173
measurements in reference to the bones 45, 109–10, 150–1
meridian clock cycle 101–3, 147
Metal
  controlled by Fire 116
  controller of Wood 116, 127
  directional number 50, 51
  element pattern 42
  Large Intestine and Lungs 51, 130, 198
  on meridian clock 102
  in nei dan meditation 200, 203
  as one of five phases 113
  opposite channel pairs 63
  pattern of channel placement 59–62
  point 117, 169
  reinforced by Earth 144, 147
  relation to po 130, 198
  right of He Tu 49, 51
  at sixth junction 41
  as Yang channel 59
  as Yin channel 58
microcosmic orbit *see* small heavenly orbit
middle dan tian 179, 181
middle layer 43–4, 69–70, 132, 142, 143, 149
Mountain 54, 55, 56, 63, 64
moxibustion 156, 157, 162
muscle channels
  conditions 106–9
  effect of anger 125
  and months of the year 104
  represented in *Ling Shu* 150
  supporting 159
  and wei qi circulation 105–6

Nan Ching 22, 117, 144
nature and humanity 17–18, 20, 113, 173
neck
  conditions 90, 91, 92, 106, 108
  middle dan tian range 179
  in nei dan meditation 185
  upper dan tian range 179
needling
  and acupuncture practice 131–3
  contra-lateral 143
  distal 148–9
  foundation method goals 155, 156
  levels of 21, 143, 148–9
  nine needles 133–4, 142–3
    channels and conditions 138
    as framework for viewing pathology 139
    names, numbers and size 134–7
  opposite 148
  order of insertion 156, 158
  technique methods 69, 151–2, 158
nei dan inner meditation
  cauldron analogy 183–4
  focusing 189
  introduction to 173–81
  lower dan tian 187–9
  preparation 184–6
  small heavenly orbit 190–5
  spiraling 189–90
  see also Five Shen Nei Dan
nourishing qi cycle 101–3, 147, 174
numbers method 52

One Cloud 174
opposite needling 148
organs
  colors 201–2
  conditions 94–7
  rejuvenation 209–10
  sensory 69, 70
  supporting 159
original qi 183–4
original spirit *see* yuan shen

paired Yin channels 42
pathogens 20, 21, 27, 28, 43, 85, 101, 103, 105–6, 110
pathways 27–40, 67–70, 158

Pericardium
  connecting channel conditions 98
  divergent channel
    distribution 63–4
    pathways 37–8
    points 77, 79–80, 84, 170
    sequence 41, 42, 51
    as Yin 64
  major channel conditions 93
  muscle channel
    conditions 109
    cycle 105
    month 104
  organ
    conditions 96
    deficiency treatment 166–8
    hour of birth 111
    nourishing qi 102
    resonances 115
    wei qi 105
    as Yin 59
plum blossom 73, 77, 156, 157, 160, 169
po 122–3
  controlled by shen 116
  controller of hun 116
  correspondences 130, 198
  group dynamics 126–7
  Lung as shelter of 115, 169
  middle dan tian 179
  as spirit of Lung 116, 168, 177, 203
primary channels *see* major channels
psychological condition 113

qi
  circulation of 151, 159
  distribution of 69
  entering and exiting 145
  excess and insufficient 91
  gathering 192–3
  needle to arouse 135, 138
  needle to capture 135
  in nei dan meditation 180, 189, 192, 195
  as one of three treasures 52, 67
  original 183–4
  rebellious 90
  regulation of 114
  sea of 187–8, 189
  source 109, 148, 150, 178, 180, 187
  spiraling 189–90

spirit 173–4
storehouse of 115
variations of 181
as vital substance 27
as Yang 174
yuan 110, 138, 180, 181, 183
see also nourishing qi cycle; wei qi
Qi Bo 173
Qi Gong 150–1, 177, 180, 187

reducing 69, 73, 85, 151–2, 169
reinforcing 69, 85, 142, 151–2, 155, 159
relationships 19–20
Ren channel 98, 102–3, 187, 190–2, 193, 195
river points 20, 144
rivers and channels 18, 149–50
roots and ends 21, 43, 85, 145–7
"Roots of Spirit" 149
Rushing Yang 34, 40

San Jiao
  connecting channel conditions 98
  divergent channel
    distribution 63–4
    pathways 37–8
    points 79–80, 84, 164, 170
    sequence 41, 42, 51
    treatment assistance 164, 167–8
    as Yang 64
  major channel conditions 93
  muscle channel
    conditions 108
    cycle 105
    month 104
  organ
    conditions 96
    hour of birth 111
    nourishing qi 102
    resonances 115
    wei qi 105
    as Yang 59
San Qing 52
sea points 20, 72, 75, 144, 165
second junction 31, 32, 41, 83
sensory organs 69, 70
separate channels *see* divergent channels
Shao Yang 40, 42, 85, 105, 146–7, 164
Shao Yin 40, 85, 105, 118, 129, 146–7, 167, 205

Shao Yong 48
shen 118–19
  controlled by zhi 116
  controller of po 116
  correspondences 130, 198
  group dynamics 126–7, 129
  and Heart 115, 116, 177, 179
  jing-qi-shen 181
  as one of three treasures 52, 67
  see also five shen
Shrinking Yin 32
sinew channels *see* muscle channels
sixth junction 39, 40, 41, 84
small heavenly orbit 190–1
  first method 191–2
  gathering qi 192–3
  nomenclature 187
  as preparation for Five Shen Nei Dan 197
  second method 193
  third method 193–5
Small Intestine
  connecting channel conditions 98
  divergent channel
    distribution 63–4
    ends and beginnings 146
    pathways 35–6
    points 77–8, 79, 84, 170
    roots and ends 85, 147
    sequence 41, 42, 51
    treatment assistance 166
    as Yang 64
  major channel conditions 92
  muscle channel
    conditions 108
    cycle 105
    month 104
  organ
    conditions 95
    correspondences 130, 198
    hour of birth 111
    innate quality 118
    nourishing qi 102
    resonances 115
    wei qi 105
    as Yang 59
  smiling into the five organs 198–9
source qi 109, 148, 150, 178, 180, 187
  see also yuan qi
space 20, 42, 101, 103, 104, 110, 120
spiraling 189–90

spirit *see* shen
Spleen
  connecting channel conditions 98
  divergent channel
    distribution 63–4
    ends and beginnings 146
    in He Tu 50–1
    pathways 33–4
    points 71, 75–6, 84, 170
    roots and ends 85, 147
    sequence 41, 42, 50, 51
    treatment assistance 144–5, 157, 159, 164–5
    as Yin 64
  emotions 116, 177, 208–9
  major channel conditions 91
  muscle channel
    conditions 107
    cycle 105
    month 104
  in nei dan meditation 174, 185, 199, 200, 201, 203, 205, 208–10
  organ
    center 184
    conditions 95
    correspondences 130, 198
    focusing attention 187
    hour of birth 111
    middle dan tian 179, 181
    nourishing qi 102
    qi 183
    resonances 115
    as storehouse 115
    wei qi 105
    as yi 116, 123–5, 127, 130, 177, 179, 198, 203
    as Yin 58, 113
spring points 20, 79, 144
stem cells 109
Stomach
  connecting channel conditions 98
  divergent channel
    distribution 63–4
    ends and beginnings 146
    in He Tu 50–1
    pathways 33–4
    points 71, 73, 75–6, 77, 79, 81, 84, 170
    roots and ends 85, 147
    sequence 41, 42, 50, 51
    treatment assistance 159, 164–5
    as Yang 64
  major channel conditions 91

Stomach *cont.*
  muscle channel
    conditions 106–7
    cycle 105
    month 104
    in nei dan meditation 201
  organ
    conditions 95
    correspondences 130, 198
    hour of birth 111
    middle dan tian 179, 181
    nourishing qi 102, 147
    resonances 115
    wei qi 105
    as Yang 59
    relation to Spleen 123, 125, 128–9, 130, 133, 144, 145, 157, 198
  stream points 20, 144, 162, 164
Su Wen 17–18, 21, 52, 113
superficial layer 43, 69–70, 73, 109–10, 132, 142, 143, 149, 150
supraclavicular dossa *see* Broken Dish
symbolism method 52

Tai Yang 40, 42, 85, 105, 146–7
Tai Yin 40, 85, 105, 136, 146–7
Taoist meditations 23
Taoist philosophy 128, 180
third junction 33, 34, 41, 84
three dan tian 177–81
three layers of the body 20–1, 142–3
  see also deep layer; middle layer; superficial layer
three treasures 22, 52, 67, 113, 181, 210
throat
  as area of ending 85, 146, 147
  conditions 90, 91, 92, 93, 94, 97, 98
  divergent channels running along 32, 34, 36, 38, 40, 69
  points 73, 75, 77, 79, 81, 83–4, 195
Thunder 54, 55, 56, 63, 64
time 20, 101, 103, 104, 105, 110–11
tongue
  conditions 93, 108
  correspondences 198
  Heart opens to 119
  middle of 84
  in nei dan meditation 202

root of 30, 34, 71, 77, 83, 84, 91
tip of 77, 84, 184
transporting points 20, 117, 141, 144–5
transverse connecting channels 99
trigrams 52–65
Triple Heater 38
tui na 135, 157, 162

unions *see* junctions
upper dan tian 179, 181, 192

Water
  controlled by Earth 116, 129
  controller of Fire 116
  converges in Bladder 115
  correspondences 128, 130, 198, 202
  directional numbers 50
  in first junction 40
  in He Tu 49, 51
  importance of 180
  on meridian clock 102
  in nei dan meditation 199–200
  as one of five phases 113
  relation to Kidney 120, 200
  relation to zhi 129, 130
  trigrams 54, 55, 56, 60–2, 63, 64
  as Yin 205
wei layer *see* superficial layer
wei qi 105–6, 110, 134, 138, 148, 150, 174
well points 20, 144, 146
Wind 54, 55, 56, 63, 64
Wood
  controlled by Metal 116, 127
  controller of Earth 116, 127
  correspondences 130, 198
  directional number 50, 51
  as Foot Yang channel 42
  Gallbladder and Liver 51
  on meridian clock 102
  in nei dan meditation 200, 202
  as one of five phases 113
  opposite channel pairs 63
  overacting 125
  position in He Tu 49, 51
  relation to hun 121
  at second junction 41
  as Yang channel 59–61
  as Yin channel 58–9, 61–2
Wu (healers) 173

Wu Ji *see* chaos
Wu Wei 118

Xiao Zhou Tien *see* small heavenly orbit

Yang channels 59–61
Yang Ming 40, 42, 85, 105, 146–7
Yang organs 152
Yang trigrams 54–5, 58, 59
yi 123–5
  controlled by hun 116
  controller of zhi 116
  correspondences 130, 198
  function of 197
  group dynamics 126, 127–9
  in nei dan meditation 199, 201, 202–3, 208–9
  relation to Spleen 115, 116, 177, 179, 187, 208–9
Yin channels 42, 58–9, 61–2, 64
Yin organs 152
Yin trigrams 54–5, 58
Yin-Yang
  channel pairs 42, 99
  and Ba Gua 57–62
  and transporting points 144–5
  in Early Heaven Ba Gua 52–5, 56–7
  in He Tu diagram 48–51
ying layer *see* middle layer
ying qi 103, 105, 138, 146, 147
yuan layer *see* deep layer
yuan qi 110, 138, 180, 181, 183
  see also source qi
yuan shen 118, 126, 130, 175, 177, 179

zang fu 89, 94
zhi 119–21
  controlled by yi 116
  controlling shen 116
  correspondences 130, 177, 198, 202
  group dynamics 126, 128–9
  relation to Kidney 115, 116, 167
zhong wan 147, 195